Laparoscopic Cholecystectomy: Problems and Solutions

To Anne and Diana,
to Christina, Joanna, Helen, Richard
and Philip, and to Rosemary

Laparoscopic Cholecystectomy
Problems and Solutions

DAVID C. DUNN MChir, FRCS
Consultant Surgeon, Department of General Surgery,
Addenbrooke's Hospital, Cambridge;
Associate Lecturer and Director of Surgical Studies,
University of Cambridge School of Clinical Medicine;
Penrose May Teacher, Royal College of Surgeons, London;
Formerly Director of Medical Studies,
St John's College, Cambridge

CHRISTOPHER J.E. WATSON FRCS
Research Registrar, Department of Surgery,
Addenbrooke's Hospital, Cambridge

OXFORD

BLACKWELL SCIENTIFIC PUBLICATIONS

LONDON EDINBURGH BOSTON

MELBOURNE PARIS BERLIN VIENNA

© 1992 by
Blackwell Scientific Publications
Editorial Offices:
Osney Mead, Oxford OX2 OEL
25 John Street, London WC1N 2BL
23 Ainslie Place, Edinburgh EH3 6AJ
3 Cambridge Center, Cambridge
    Massachusetts 02142, USA
54 University Street, Carlton
    Victoria 3053, Australia

Other Editorial Offices:
Librairie Arnette SA
2, rue Casimir-Delavigne
75006 Paris
France

Blackwell Wissenschafts-Verlag
Meinekestrasse 4
D-1000 Berlin 15
Germany

Blackwell MZV
Feldgasse 13
A-1238 Wien
Austria

First published 1992

Set by Alden Multimedia Ltd,
Northampton
Printed in Great Britain at the
Alden Press, Oxford, and bound
at the Green Street Bindery, Oxford

DISTRIBUTORS

Marston Book Services Ltd
PO Box 87
Oxford OX2 ODT
(*Orders*: Tel: 0865 791155
          Fax: 0865 791927
          Telex: 837515)

USA
Blackwell Scientific Publications, Inc.
3 Cambridge Center
Cambridge, MA 02142
(*Orders*: Tel: 800 759-6102
          617 225-0401)

Canada
  Times Mirror
  Professional Publishing, Ltd
  5240 Finch Avenue East
  Scarborough, Ontario M1S 5A2
  (*Orders*: Tel: 800 268-4178
            416 298-1588)

Australia
  Blackwell Scientific Publications
  (Australia) Pty Ltd
  54 University Street
  Carlton, Victoria 3053
  (*Orders*: Tel: 03 347-0300)

A catalogue record for this book
is available from the British Library

0-632-03444-0

Contents

Preface, x

Acknowledgements, xi

Introduction, xii

1 Insufflation and optical equipment, 1
Verres needle, 1
Cannulae, 1
Trocars, 3
Hasson cork cannula, 5
Laparoscopes, 6
   Standard laparoscope, 6
   Operating laparoscope, 6
Video system, 8
   Light cable, 8
   Light source, 8
   Camera, 9
   Television monitors, 9
   Video recorder/printer, 10
Insufflator, 10
Laparoscope warmer, 13

2 Hand instruments, 15
Coagulating instruments, 15
   Diathermy hook, 15
   Diathermy spade, 15
   Diathermy button probe, 15
Scissors, 16
   Microscissors, 17
   Hooked scissors, 17
   Plain scissors, 17
Holding/grasping forceps, 17
   Self-holding devices, 17
   Grasping/holding mechanisms, 19
   Jaw types, 20
Needle holders, 20
Dissecting instruments, 21
Suction/irrigation devices, 22
Sutures, 24
Clip appliers, 24
Specialized instruments, 26
   Reddick–Olsen cholangiography clamp, 26
   Cholangiography catheter, 26
   Dormia basket, 26

3 Lasers and laparoscopic surgery, 28
What is a laser? 28

Production of laser energy, 29
Properties of laser light, 30
Pulsed and continuous-wave mode lasers, 30
Laser–tissue interactions, 30
Dangers of lasers, 31
Characteristics of different lasers, 31
Delivery of laser light, 33
Contact lasers, 33

4 Laparoscopic techniques, 35
Converting to laparoscopic operative techniques, 35
Producing a pneumoperitoneum, 37
Safety tests, 38
Initial laparoscopy, 40
Retraction, 41
Abdominal wall, 41
Gallbladder, 41
Falciform lift, 41
Inserting an extra port, 42
Dissection/haemostasis, 42
Using the diathermy hook, 42
Dissecting scissors, 44
Using the laser, 45
Blunt dissection, 46
Suction and irrigation, 47
Clips, 47
Multifire clip applicator, 48
Self-locking clips, 48
Tying knots and suturing, 49
External knotting (Roeder knot), 49
Preformed catgut ligature, 50
Suturing, 52
Internal knots, 53

5 Pre-operative preparation, 56
History and examination, 56
Investigations, 57
Ultrasound, 57
Oral cholecystogram, 57
Liver function tests, 57
Endoscopic cholangiography, 58
Intravenous cholangiography, 58
Patient preparation, 58
Laxative suppositories, 58
Shaving, 58
Premedication, 59
Bladder emptying, 59
Deep vein thrombosis prophylaxis, 59

Antibiotic prophylaxis, 59
Informed consent, 60
  Possibility of open cholecystectomy, 60
  Choledocholithiasis, 60
  Video tapes, 60
  Recovery, 60

6 Anaesthesia for laparoscopic cholecystectomy, 61
M.J. LINDOP
Pre-operative management, 61
  General, 61
  Premedication, 61
Operative management, 62
  Bradycardia, 62
  Heat loss, 62
  Muscle relaxation, 63
  Raised intra-abdominal pressure, 63
  Potential for gas embolus, 64
  Potential for haemorrhage, 64
  Gastric distension, 65
  Bladder, 65
  Position and patient safety, 65
  Other drugs, 65
Postoperative management, 65
  Wound pain, 66
  Shoulder pain, 66
  Nausea, 66
  Shivering, 67
Summary of key features of anaesthetic management, 67

7 The operation of laparoscopic cholecystectomy, 68
Anatomy, 68
  Normal anatomy, 68
  Important variations in anatomy, 69
Setting up, 74
  Position of patient, 74
  Layout of theatre, 76
  Setting up theatre, 76
  Preparation of the skin, 78
  Sterile connections, 78
  Testing routines, 79
The operation, 80
  Inserting the operative ports, 80
  Exposure of Calot's triangle, 85
  Retraction of the gallbladder, 85
  Adhesions to the gallbladder, 86
  Defining the cystic duct, 87

Cholangiogram, 88
The cystic artery, 91
Freeing the gallbladder from its bed, 92
The gallbladder bed, 93
Inserting a drain, 93
Haemostasis, 94
Peritoneal toilet, 95
Extracting the gallbladder, 95
Use of a bag for extraction, 96
Enlarging the exit port, 97
Closing the linea alba, 97
Closing the skin, 98

8 Stones in the hepatic and common bile ducts, 100
The problem, 100
Methods of management, 100
Stones found before operation, 100
Stones found during operation, 101
Laparoscopic techniques for bile duct exploration, 101
Exploration under X-ray control, 102
Exploration through a choledochotomy, 105
Exploration using a flexible choledochoscope, 106
Laparoscopic lithotripsy of common duct stones, 107

9 Dealing with operative difficulties, 108
Technical problems, 108
Loss of vision, 108
Fogging of laparoscope, 109
Obesity, 110
Loss of pneumoperitoneum, 112
Haemorrhage, 112
Bleeding from ports, 112
Retroperitoneal haematoma, 113
Major haemorrhage into the peritoneal cavity, origin unclear, 114
Major haemorrhage from hepatic or cystic arteries, or portal vein, 114
Haemorrhage from the gallbladder bed, 115
Problems due to inflammation and fibrosis, 116
Peritoneal adhesions, 116
Adherent duodenum and colon, 119
Small shrunken gallbladder, 119
Empyema of the gallbladder, 120
Fibrosis around the portal triad, 120
Oedematous thickened gallbladder wall, 121
Problems due to surgical trauma, 121
Verres needle or trocar injuries, 121
Damage to the bowel, 121
Damage to hepatic or common bile ducts, 122
Hole in the gallbladder, 123

Loss of stones in the peritoneum, 123
CO$_2$ embolism, 124
Loss of a needle in the peritoneal cavity, 124
Anatomical and pathological difficulties, 125
Distended gallbladder, 125
Intrahepatic gallbladder, 125
Abnormal anatomy, 126
Stones in the cystic duct, 126
Stones in the common bile duct, 127
Short cystic duct, 127
Wide cystic duct, 127
Large stones, 128
Difficult extraction, 128
Collapse of patient, 129

10 Postoperative course, 130
Pain, 130
Analgesia, 131
Oro-gastric tube, 131
Urinary catheter, 131
Drains, 131
Oral fluids, 131
Oral feeding, 132
Mobility and convalescence, 132
Follow-up, 132

Appendix: Handout for patients, 133

Index, 137

Preface

Having learned the technique of laparoscopic cholecystectomy, the authors found they had to assimilate a great deal of information from a wide variety of sources. Both are now involved in training others to undertake this technique and began to feel there was a need to put all this information together into a succinct textbook which would be of value to those who were also learning. This book is the result. It deals in a basic and didactic way with the technology and instrumentation required, and the steps and problems of the operation itself. It is designed to be of value to surgeons learning laparoscopic cholecystectomy, and to junior medical staff and medical students. It will also fill a need for information required by theatre and ward nurses, and general practitioners.

Acknowledgements

The authors are indebted to numerous surgeons from several countries who passed on their enthusiasm for this new form of surgery and gave us advice and help, both in person and through published papers and books. These include Dr Joe Petelin who taught the senior author the basic technique, Professor Alfred Cuschieri and Dr Tehemton Udwadia. We would never have been able to start the operation in Cambridge without the unfailing help of Richard Koronowski and numerous representatives and sales managers from various equipment, instrument, and suture companies, including Ethicon, Auto Suture, Sigmacon, and Wolf. We are grateful to our initial patients for having the courage to let us try this new operation for them. The enormous patience, tolerance, enthusiasm and professionalism of the theatre staff at Addenbrooke's Hospital and The Evelyn Hospital, Cambridge, are much appreciated as is the support of our anaesthetic colleagues, particularly Dr M. Lindop who also contributed Chapter 6. Finally Ros Britton has typed innumerable versions of the manuscript under extreme time pressure and nothing would have been produced without her help.

Introduction

One of the fruits of the communication and technology revolution has been the extraordinary spread of laparoscopic cholecystectomy as a replacement for open cholecystectomy for the treatment of gallstones. Early in 1990 neither of the present authors had heard of laparoscopic cholecystectomy. Following a talk by Alfred Cuschieri of Dundee in March 1990 attempts to get the operation started locally were met with disbelief and comments such as 'anyone with any sense would have their gallbladder removed the proper way, through a large abdominal incision'. At that time, only a handful of people around the world had performed more than 50 such procedures. Following painstaking and pioneering work in laparoscopic techniques by Semm, the first operation was carried out by Mouret in 1987, and Dubois published the first series of 60 cases in December 1989. As this book is being written in December 1991 many thousands of such operations have been carried out throughout the world and surgeons everywhere are taking up the new technique with enthusiasm.

What has caused this excitement amongst surgeons? The answer is the same factor that has stimulated surgical endeavour through the ages — the alleviation of suffering in patients. Suddenly, surgeons have been confronted with a technique that can relieve the suffering inflicted by gallstones at a far less cost in patient suffering due to the operation itself.

Surgery has always been about inflicting damage to achieve a cure. The profession has steadily worked towards minimizing the trauma inflicted while still achieving its therapeutic goals. Haemostasis, asepsis and anaesthesia were all steps along this road. Minimal access surgery is the next step and its value has already been proven in gynaecology, urology and orthopaedics. In order for intraperitoneal minimal access surgery to become routine, there had to be major technological advances especially in video equipment. This allowed the surgeon to operate by remote control within the closed abdominal cavity. The operations to be performed were delicate and close to major abdominal structures, so visual discrimination had to be sufficient to minimize the risks of serious damage. The space age produced such technology, and enthusiasts for laparoscopy, struggling for years with inadequate vision and instrumentation, grasped the opportunity and showed the world what could be done.

In March 1990, one of us (DCD) set out to institute a general surgical laparoscopic service in Cambridge based on 17 years of consultant practice in conventional surgery. The other author (CJEW) was previously his registrar and was working as a research fellow at that time. In starting laparoscopic surgery, both have had to learn completely new ways of operating. They have also learned to handle equipment previously unknown to them. This includes the apparatus necessary to induce a pneumoperitoneum, video cameras and screens, irrigation and suction equipment, innumerable new instruments, a better understanding of diathermy in closed spaces and the whole new world of lasers in surgery. In doing this, they had to glean information from a wide variety of sources and teachers (the most important of which are mentioned in the acknowledgements). Much of the written information was presented in a form which was difficult to comprehend. Information about solving many of the problems we encountered simply was not written down anywhere.

While laparoscopic surgery is still in its infancy, we find ourselves teaching others how to set up such a service and to perform laparoscopic cholecystectomies safely. In doing so, we constantly find ourselves answering the same questions, questions which trainee surgeons are no doubt asking all over the world. We therefore felt we should put our new found, if very incomplete, knowledge down on paper and at least offer it to others to ease their way along the path we have recently trod. To experts in the field much we have written will seem simplistic and obvious. Our only excuse is that it is what we found difficult and it is what our trainees ask us now. We hope it will be of value to others. It would also be surprising if there are not some mistakes and misunderstandings in what we have written. We hope our readers will be kind enough to point these out to us as we are still anxious to learn as much as possible about this exciting form of surgery.

1: Insufflation and optical equipment

Verres needle
Cannulae
Trocars
Hasson cork cannula
Laparoscopes
   Standard laparoscope
   Operating laparoscope

Video system
   Light cable
   Light source
   Camera
   Television monitors
   Video recorder/printer
Insufflator
Laparoscope warmer

Verres needle

The instrument

The Verres needle is used for the initial creation of the pneumoperitoneum. It comprises a long, sharp needle, through the centre of which passes a blunt spring-loaded hollow trocar (Fig. 1.1). Gas flows through this central trocar and out of a side hole at its end. The spring mechanism allows the blunt central trocar to shield the cutting edge of the needle until it meets resistance, at which point the trocar is pushed back. The trocar remains retracted while the needle is pushed through the abdominal wall, to spring back and shield the needle once resistance disappears in the peritoneal cavity. The other end of the needle has a luer lock inlet for attachment of the insufflation tubing, and a manual on/off tap.

Notes

The patency of the needle and function of the spring safety mechanism should be verified each time it is used (see Chapter 7, p. 80). Patency may be compromised by obstruction of the small terminal gas outflow port.

Cannulae

The instrument

A cannula is a tube of fixed internal diameter through which instruments are introduced into the peritoneal cavity. At one end is a rubber gasket providing a gas tight seal around the instruments. The cannula is sealed by either a spring-loaded trumpet valve or flap valve mechanism at the outer end (Fig. 1.2). The valve occludes the lumen completely to prevent gas leaks when no instrument is in place. The cannula may also have a luer lock attachment for the insufflation gas.

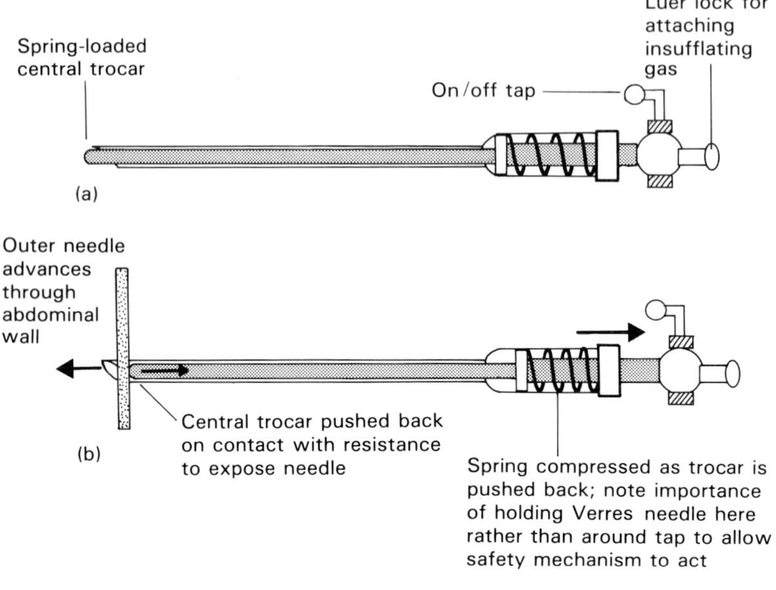

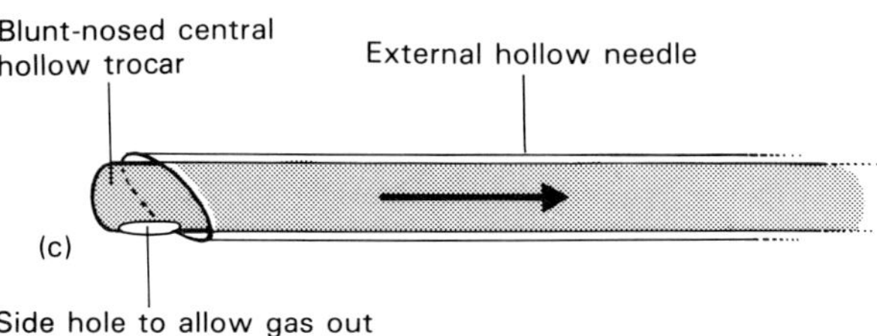

Fig. 1.1 The Verres needle. Diagrams to show the mechanism of action.

The internal diameters vary according to manufacturer, and are essentially either small (5–6 mm) or large (10–12 mm).

Notes

1 It is important to use the correct size of instrument (compatible with the cannula) to prevent gas leaks. Reducing sleeves and diaphragms are available to reduce the effective internal diameter of the cannula.

2 Inspect the rubber port cover or diaphragm regularly. It can be cut by the trocar or other instrument causing a gas leak.

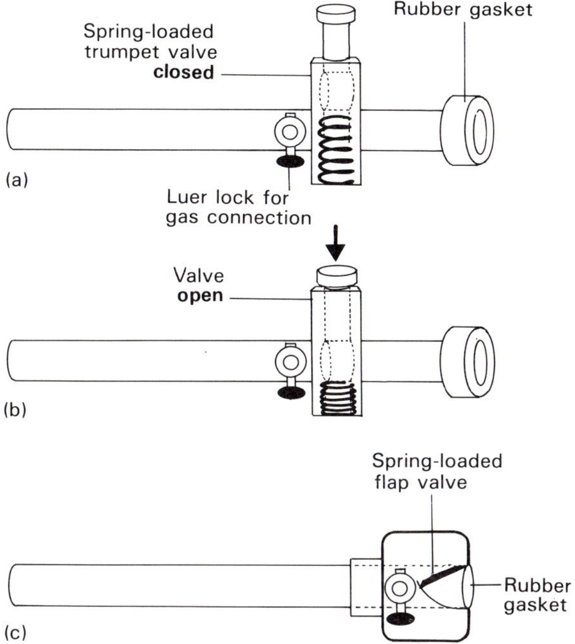

Fig. 1.2 Basic cannulae for laparoscopy. Escape of gas may be prevented by a trumpet valve or a spring-loaded flap valve. The rubber gasket fits snugly around the shaft of instruments.

Trocars

The instrument

The trocar passes through the cannula centre providing a sharp point to facilitate passage through the abdominal wall. Two styles of point are available, conical and pyramidal (Fig. 1.3). The pyramidal

Fig. 1.3 Two types of trocar point. (a) Pyramidal point; (b) conical point.

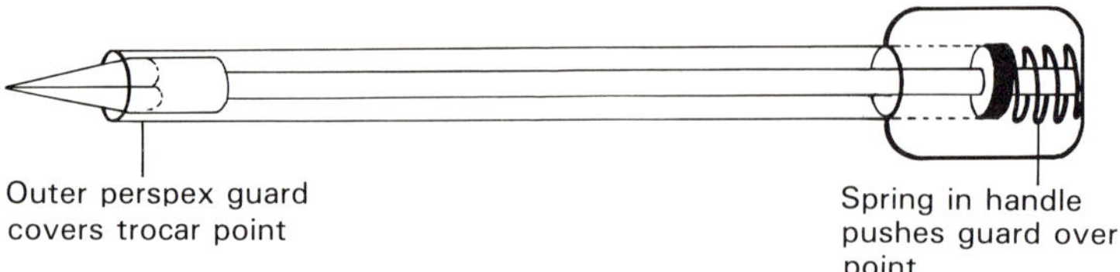

Fig. 1.4 Guarded trocar point (disposable) cannulae often have a guard which springs forward once the instrument is in the peritoneal cavity.

point is a more effective cutting point, but can also cut neighbouring vessels in the abdominal wall.

Notes

The trocar passes with equal facility through vessels and viscera. A variety of disposable cannulae are available with shielded trocars, in which the shield retracts once on passage through the abdominal wall, and is then locked to guard the trocar point (Fig. 1.4). This reduces the risk of injury to intraperitoneal structures, and this type of cannula is recommended for the primary puncture site.

Danger

The guard does not shoot forward until it is free of resistance (Fig. 1.5). If the peritoneum is loose and moves ahead of the trocar tip, it is possible to puncture both the peritoneum and a nearby vessel against the posterior abdominal wall.

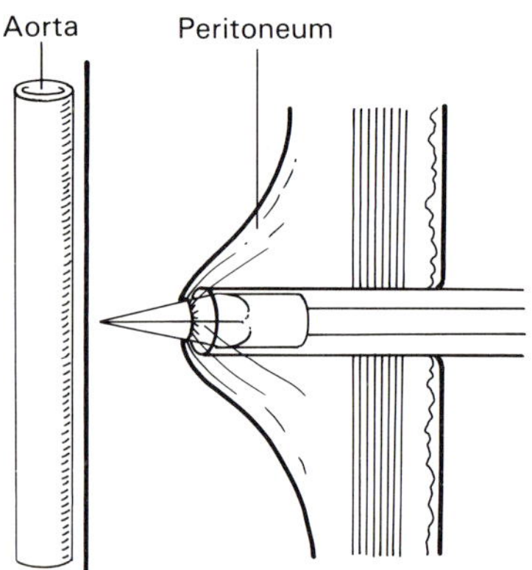

Fig. 1.5 The guard does not spring forward until it is free of peritoneum.

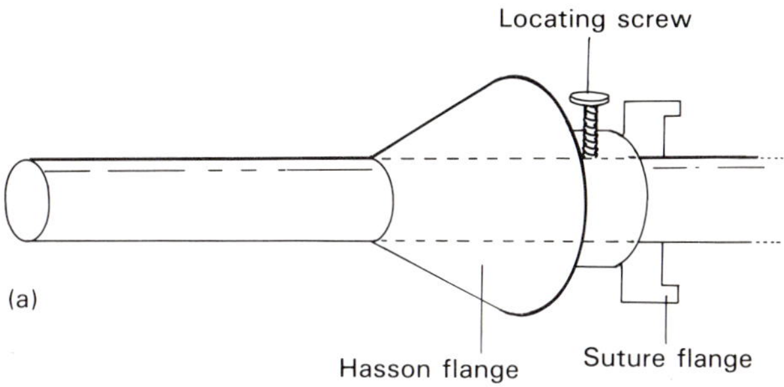

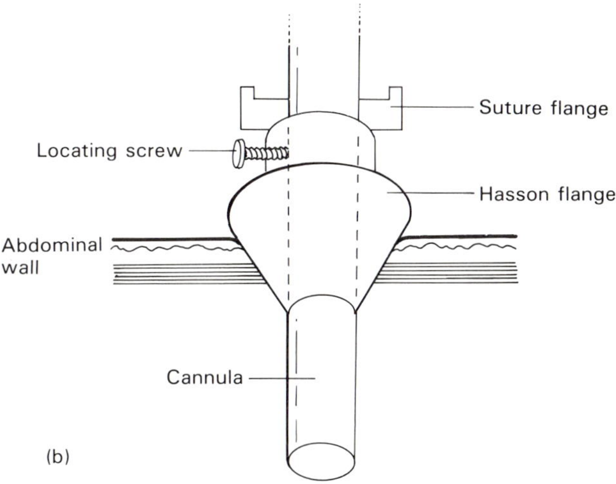

Fig. 1.6 The Hasson 'cork' cannula.

Hasson cork cannula

The instrument

The Hasson cannula (Fig. 1.6) has a conical flange on the outside and is suitable for use when a cutdown approach has been made for initial cannulation. It can then be inserted under direct vision. Originally developed to slide over a standard cannula, it is now also made as an integral unit. The cannula should be held or sutured down against the edges of the incision in the abdominal wall, like a cork in a bottle. Some flanges have a screw thread.

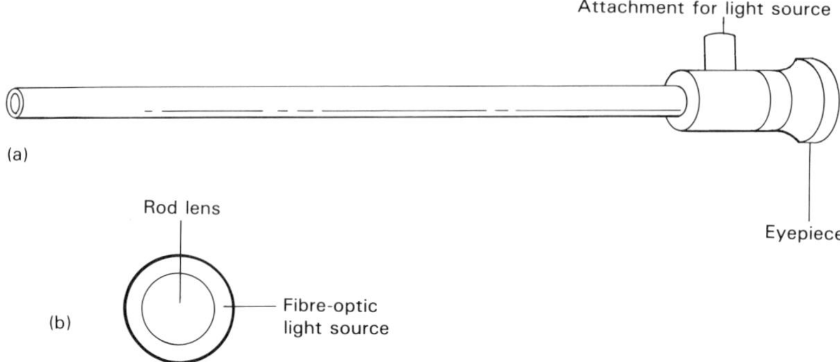

Fig. 1.7 The standard laparoscope consists of (a) a central rod lens system surrounded by (b) optical fibres for transmission of light.

Laparoscopes

Standard laparoscope

The instrument
The central core of the laparoscope is the Hopkins rod–lens system (Fig. 1.7). This solid lens system focuses and transmits light from the abdomen back to the eyepiece. Around this central core is a sheath of optical fibres carrying light into the abdomen from an attachment on the side of the laparoscope. The laparoscope may be forward viewing or view slightly off centre (25 or 30°). Laparoscopes vary in diameter from 5 to 12 mm. A 10 mm scope transmits four times as much light as a 5 mm scope and hence gives a better view. It is the minimum required for safe laparoscopic cholecystectomy.

Notes
The 25/30° laparoscope allows the observer to view around obstructions such as distended viscera (Fig. 1.8). This can be particularly useful during laparoscopic cholecystectomy when the view of Calot's triangle is obscured by bowel, liver or omental fat. Rotation of the scope allows vision upwards and downwards and to left and right.

Operating laparoscope

The instrument
An operating laparoscope is a 10 mm instrument with a smaller (e.g. 5 mm) operating channel down its centre along which instruments may be passed, to lie along the axis of vision (Fig. 1.9).

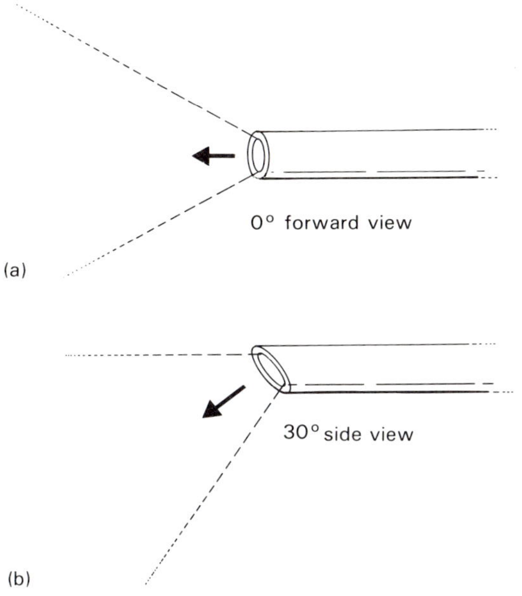

Fig. 1.8 o and 30° viewing laparoscopes.

Notes
1 The operating channel restricts the view, which is comparable to that of the smaller 5 mm laparoscope.
2 The operating channel is limited in its usefulness, and a separate second puncture site gives greater manipulative potential, though an extra scar.

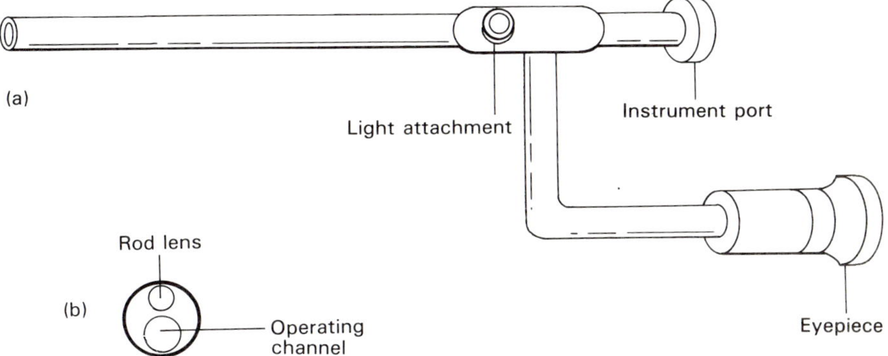

Fig. 1.9 The operating laparoscope.

Video system

The video system comprises the light cable, the light source and the camera.

Light cable

The instrument

The light cable consists of a sheath of fine optical fibres which carry the light from source to laparoscope. On each end is an appropriate adaptor for connection to light source and laparoscope.

Notes

1 Individual fibres are easily broken, reducing light transmission. The cable should not be bent, but rather allowed to take up its natural curve.

2 When starting the operation and draping the patient, be careful to pass out the correct end of the light cable. It is easy to desterilize the laparoscope attachment.

3 Inspection of the cable should be performed regularly. Hold one end pointing towards a light source. The other end will light with grey or black spots at the end. These spots represent broken optical fibres. If more than a quarter of the surface is lost, the cable needs replacing.

Light source

The instrument

A high intensity cold light source such as xenon or a halide is required to provide sufficient light. Losses of up to 90% of transmitted light energy are common *en route* from source to abdomen, and less powerful sources are inadequate. Large losses occur at each inter-face, as well as in the cable and laparoscope.

Notes

If there is a lot of free blood in the peritoneum the amount of reflected light is much reduced, reducing visibility. Regular irrigation and aspiration will help to maximize illumination by increasing reflected light.

Camera

The instrument

The camera attaches over the laparoscope eyepiece and in some cases is an integral part of the laparoscope. Cameras vary in sensitivity and image definition according to the number of silicon chips; a single chip camera has a resolution of 450 lines per inch, while a three chip resolves to 700 lines per inch. The basic camera chip detects black and white. Colour is achieved by pulsing light through a trichromatic filter system, and then decoding the returning image into its colour components.

Automatic adjustment of light output according to the incident light intensity detected by the camera can be achieved by an automatic iris shutter. While avoiding glare, a slow response time can be awkward, and a manual override is essential.

In order to produce an accurate spectrum of colours the camera system must be 'white balanced', that is, exposed to pure white light which is then taken as the reference value. While some cameras are able to white balance automatically, it must be manually performed in others. This simply involves pointing the laparoscope at a pure white image such as a surgical swab.

Notes

1 While in use, condensation forms on the lens of the camera resulting in misting of the image. The camera to laparoscope couple must be thoroughly dried. A ventilated couple would avoid this.
2 The camera should not be autoclaved, but rather sterilized in a suitable solution.
3 Rotation of the camera rotates the image. A square-bodied camera is easier to keep orientated than one with a round body.

Television monitors

A high resolution monitor should be compatible with the camera. For a single chip camera a standard 400 lines per inch monitor is adequate. However, to benefit from the increased resolution afforded by a three chip camera, a higher resolution monitor is required to display at around 700 lines per inch.

The larger the monitor, the clearer the image, and a 13 inch screen is a minimum requirement. The size quoted is the diagonal length of the screen, so a 15 inch screen would be 9 inches tall and 12 inches wide.

Video recorder/printer

Important for documentation, teaching and learning, these must be compatible with the camera system.

Insufflator

The instrument

The insufflator is the machine which pumps the gas into the peritoneal cavity. The first generation gynaecology insufflators delivered 1 litre of gas per minute, adequate only for short diagnostic procedures involving single ports. Laparoscopic surgery, involving three or four ports, requires faster gas delivery, since losses around ports and during instrument changes are significantly greater. Adequate insufflation is essential to create the space in which to see and operate and current generation insufflators deliver up to 8 litres per minute (Fig. 1.10).

Carbon dioxide is the gas of choice for insufflation. Alternatives such as oxygen and air carry a high risk of embolism and support combustion. Nitrous oxide has an unpredictable and uncontrollable absorption rate from the peritoneum. It also supports combustion. Carbon dioxide, however, is rapidly soluble in blood, reducing risks of gas embolism; it also suppresses combustion. The amount of absorbed carbon dioxide can be monitored indirectly from the end-tidal CO_2 level measured by the anaesthetist (see Chapter 6). The blood level of CO_2 can be controlled by alteration of the ventilation depth and rate.

Safe insufflation demands accurate monitoring of intraperitoneal pressure, and flow rate. In addition, a record of the volume of gas insufflated is particularly useful at the start of the operation. For laparoscopic surgery, the intraperitoneal pressure should be between 10 and 15 mmHg which represents a volume of 2.5–4 litres in the relaxed peritoneal cavity. Higher pressures predispose to venous compression, gas embolus, ventilatory impairment, and haemodynamic instability. The insufflator should have an automatic alarm if the pressure rises dangerously high. Lower pressures provide inadequate pneumoperitoneum. Blind insertion of the first cannula should

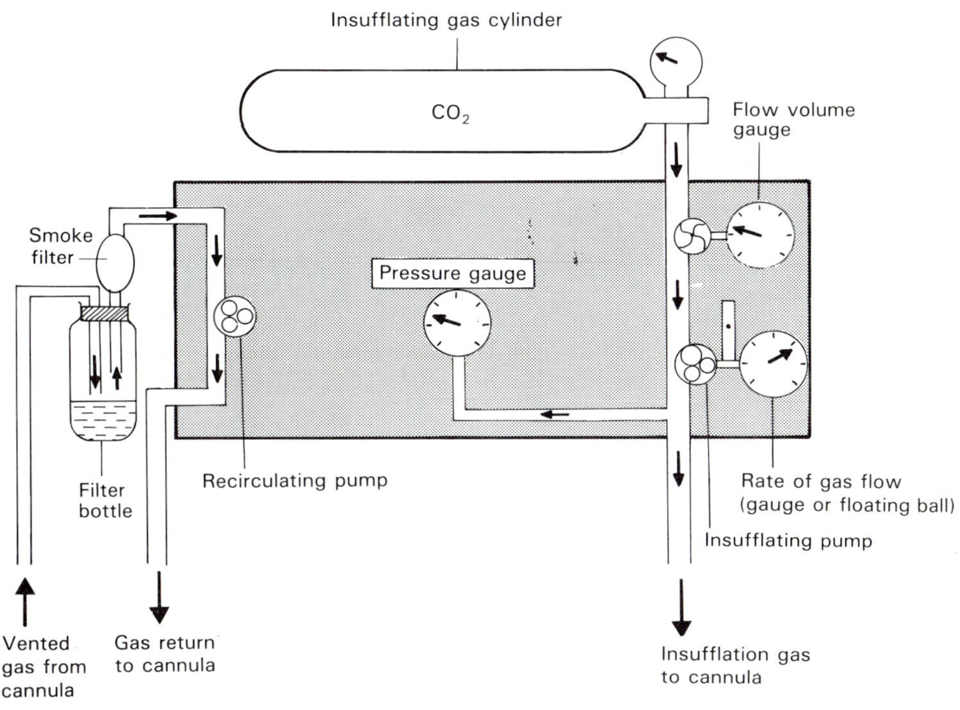

Fig. 1.10 Diagrammatic representation of an insufflator together with a smoke extraction circuit.

not be performed until at least 3 litres of gas has been insufflated, to reduce the risk to underlying bowel and mesentery.

Some insufflators have additional pumps (vents) which recirculate the gas and remove smoke and laser plume, improving the visibility.

We recommend that the output and input lines of the venting circuit should be connected to different ports to the main insufflator. In some machines the vent return and the insufflator's gas input lines join at a T-piece. This may lead to false and dangerous readings of intra-abdominal pressure. For example, if the vent return and gas input are joined end-to-end in line the insufflator records a high line pressure and cuts out irrespective of the actual intraperitoneal pressure (see Fig. 1.11). Similarly, if the gas input joins the vent return end-to-side as in Fig. 1.11 the Venturi effect results in a low pressure reading in the gas input line, again regardless of the true intraperitoneal pressure. In this configuration the result will be a

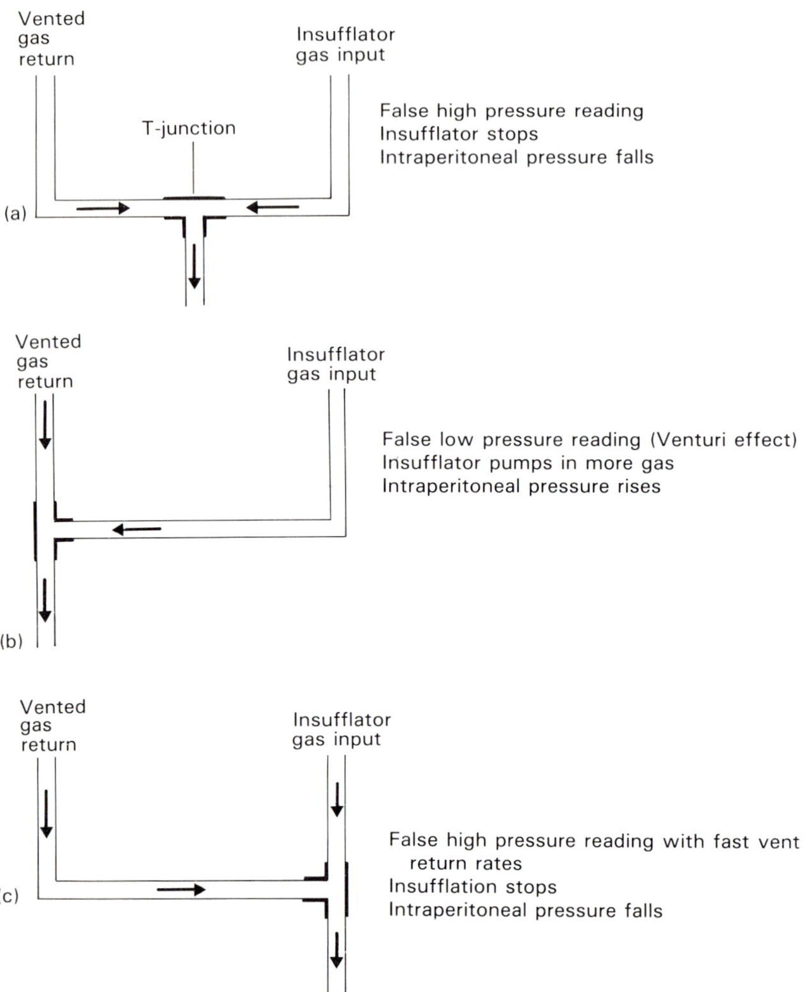

Fig. 1.11 Problems can be created by joining the vent gas return to the main insufflator input of gas (Venturi effect).

dangerously high abdominal pressure as the insufflator continues to pump.

Notes

1 At the start of each operation, the insufflation circuit should be checked for air leaks. If present they can lead to false pressure readings and misleading flow–volume readings. If a venting system

is available for smoke extraction, external air can be sucked in through a leak in this circuit.

2 High pressure may be due to a kinked insufflation tube, incomplete penetration of the cannula or Verres needle into the abdomen, external compression on the abdomen, or active contraction of abdominal muscles due to inadequate anaesthesia.

3 High flow rates or large insufflation volumes may be due to a disconnected insufflation tube, an open cannula or gas port, or leakage around a small size instrument in a large cannula.

Laparoscope warmer

The instrument

When a cold laparoscope enters the warm humid environment inside the peritoneal cavity condensation forms on the lens. This may be overcome by either pre-warming the laparoscope to body temperature, or coating the lens with a weak detergent which lowers surface tension and prevents the condensation build up. Our laparoscope warmer consists of a container of sterile water maintained at 40°C by partial immersion in a water bath (see Fig. 1.12). The 40°C setting is chosen so that the scope is still above 37° by the time it is replaced inside the abdomen. The laparoscope may be washed in this periodically to remove blood and debris during the course of the operation.

Notes

1 We use a blood warmer reset to 40°C, into which we place a bottle

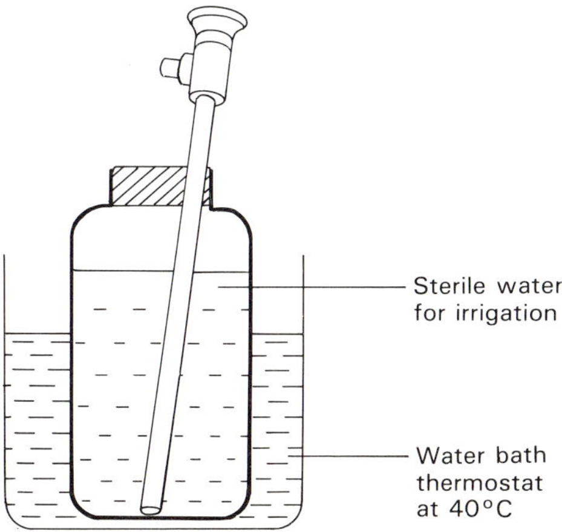

Fig. 1.12 Diagram of our laparoscope warming apparatus.

of 'sterile water for irrigation'. If this adaptation is used the blood warmer must be clearly marked 'NOT FOR BLOOD' and stored separately to avoid inadvertent use to warm blood, which it may in fact lyse.

2 The laparoscope should be placed lens down in the warm bottle of water after sterilization for at least 10 minutes before surgery to allow it to warm up.

2: Hand instruments

Coagulating instruments
  Diathermy hook
  Diathermy spade
  Diathermy button probe
Scissors
  Microscissors
  Hooked scissors
  Plain scissors
Holding/grasping forceps
  Self-holding devices
  Grasping/holding mechanisms
  Jaw types

Needle holders
Dissecting instruments
Suction/irrigation devices
Sutures
Clip appliers
Specialized instruments
  Reddick–Olsen cholangiography
    clamp
  Cholangiography catheter
  Dormia basket

Introduction

Most instruments have one of the following principle functions.

1 Coagulating instruments.

2 Scissors.

3 Holding/grasping forceps.

4 Dissecting instruments.

5 Suction/irrigation devices.

Many laparoscopic instruments perform more than one of these functions. For example, any instrument with an insulated shaft can conduct diathermy current, and be used for coagulation.

Coagulating instruments

Diathermy hook

This is probably the most useful single instrument. It has an insulated shaft ending in a right-angled bare metal point (Fig. 2.1a). This hook end allows tissue to be hooked and lifted away from surrounding tissue before being cauterized ('Hook, look, cook'; see Chapter 4, p. 43). The flat end can also be used directly on tissue to produce a wider area of coagulation.

Diathermy spade

This has a flat spade end useful for separating tissues (Fig. 2.1c), but lacks the ability to lift the tissue clear of its surroundings prior to cautery.

Diathermy button probe

The diathermy probe has an insulated shaft with a bare metal

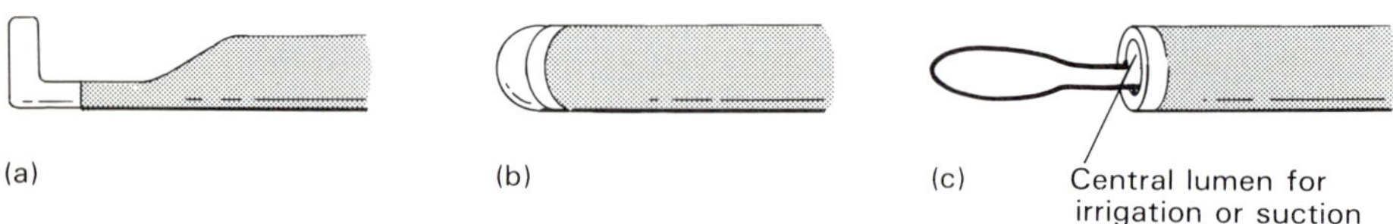

Fig. 2.1 The ends of some diathermy instruments.

rounded end (Fig. 2.1b). This transmits a diffuse diathermy current ideal for coagulation of small oozing areas in the gallbladder bed. Because of the broader contact area, it usually requires more power or more prolonged application to achieve satisfactory haemostasis.

Notes

All of the above specialized diathermy instruments have insulation down to their tips, so reducing the risk of inadvertent burning of adjacent tissues. Such burning is common when scissors or grasping forceps are used to cauterize, since the operating surgeon watching the TV image lacks depth perception and fails to perceive the proximity of the bare shaft to neighbouring tissue. Indeed the commonest cause of the apparent failure of an insulated instrument to cauterize is an inadvertent burn elsewhere.

Beware of using a diathermy current together with irrigating fluid. The current can be conducted through the fluid to produce unexpected burns elsewhere.

The tip of a diathermy instrument remains hot after the current is switched off. A hole can be made in neighbouring bowel if the probe is allowed to rest on it.

Scissors

While the hook is the most useful cutting instrument, scissors are important where diathermy is contraindicated, such as in opening the cystic duct. All scissors have one fixed blade in the axis of the

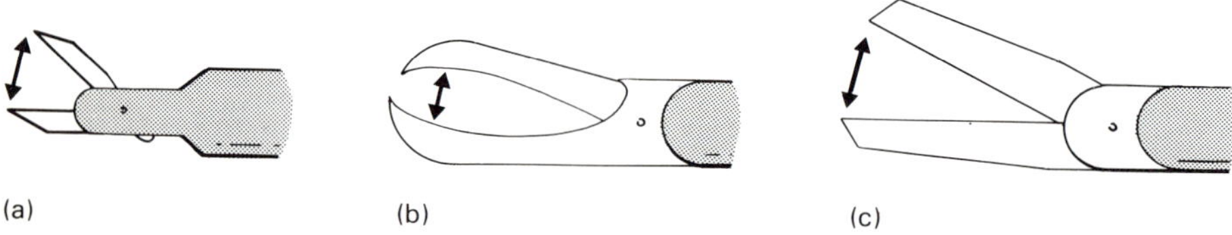

Fig. 2.2 Laparoscopic scissors.

instrument, and one moving blade. The tissue to be cut should be opposed against the fixed blade before closing the free blade onto it.

Microscissors
The fine pointed scissors, either flat or curved (Fig. 2.2a), are useful for accurate small cuts.

Hooked scissors
The hooked tips (Fig. 2.2b) allow the surgeon to see the tips in contact, and enable tissue to be lifted away from neighbouring structures before cutting, thus preventing accidental damage. They also hold tissue preventing it from rolling out of the jaws when being cut.

Plain scissors
General purpose scissors (Fig. 2.2c), useful for dissection as well as cutting and electrocautery (if insulated).

Note
Insulated scissors are rapidly blunted if used to cauterize tissue in their open jaws before cutting it.

Holding/grasping forceps
There are several different designs of grasping and holding instruments. They may be insulated or not; they may incorporate a self-holding device in their handle or have a plain handle; or they may have telescopic or hinged jaws.

Self-holding devices
Holding and grasping instruments are characterized by one fixed handle connected to the shaft of the instrument, while the other handle is connected to a central piston running through the centre of the shaft (Fig. 2.3). When the handles are squeezed the central piston moves relative to the shaft, opening or closing the blades/jaws of the instrument. To facilitate holding tissue within the jaws for a period of time, the handle incorporates a self-holding device, such as a spring or ratchet.

A spring clip on the handle holds the jaws closed but does not give a secure grip and tissue may slip from the jaws. However, the spring can be disengaged to allow more freedom of movement during dissection.

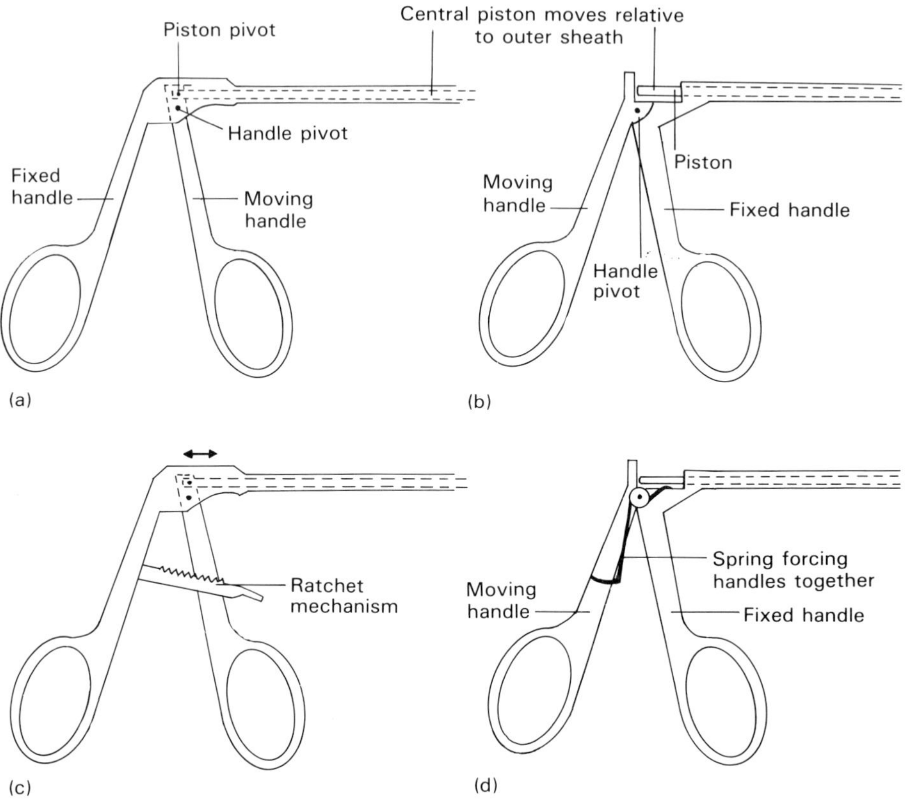

Fig. 2.3 Different types of instrument handles.

A ratchet holds the jaws closed or semi-closed in the position in which they were applied. It is particularly useful for holding the gallbladder fundus or Hartmann's pouch, maintaining its grip for as long as required.

Telescopic spring. The spring which retracts the jaws of telescopic-grasping forceps is usually quite strong, but of limited usefulness.

Notes
Self-holding devices can inhibit active manipulation of the instrument and for this reason a device which can be disengaged is particularly useful.

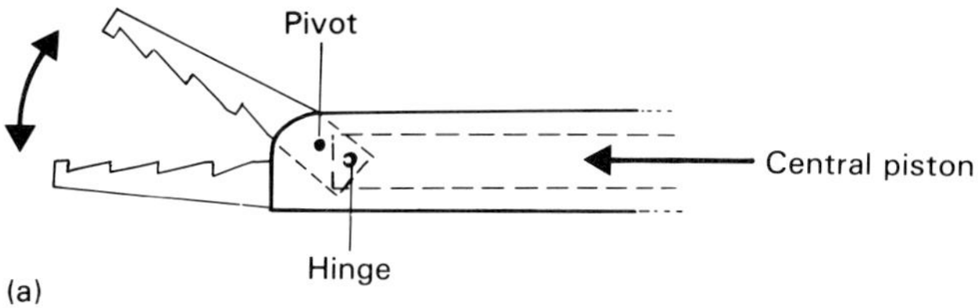

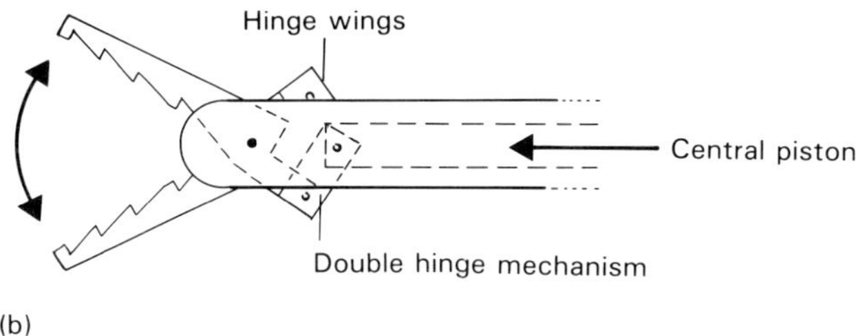

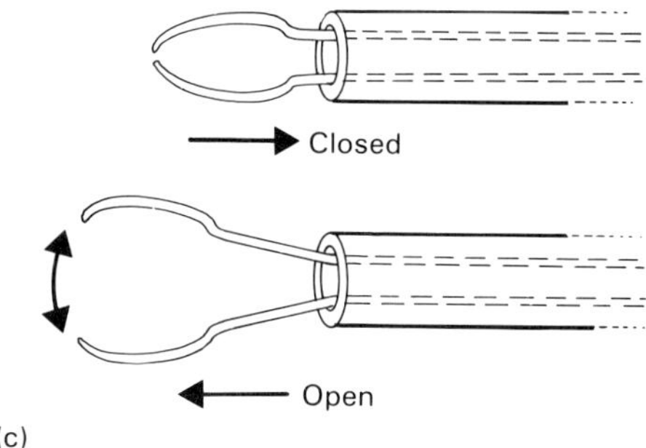

Fig. 2.4 Holding and grasping mechanisms.

Grasping/holding mechanisms (Fig. 2.4)

Telescopic-grasping mechanism

These instruments (Fig. 2.4c) have three or four jaws which splay out to grasp tissue and are spring loaded to come together when retracted back into their sheath. They can be useful to grasp a tubular structure such as a fallopian tube.

Notes

These are difficult to apply. The jaws retract away from the tissue when you are attempting to apply them.

Single jaw mechanism

These forceps have one fixed blade with the other moving against it, like scissors (Fig. 2.4a). These have a limited open angle in which to grasp tissue, and, just as with the scissors, the tissue must be opposed to the fixed jaw before the moving one is closed on it.

Double jaw mechanism

These forceps are hinged such that both jaws move, enabling more tissue to be grasped (Fig. 2.4b). This double-hinged mechanism is also better for blunt dissection.

Notes

The mechanism requires one double hinge per blade, resulting in wings protruding on either side of the shaft. These wings can jam inside a cannula if opened inside or retracted into it, and may be broken this way.

Jaw types (Fig. 2.5)

All grasping/holding forceps can damage the tissue they hold. Those with the surest grip also tend to cause the most damage, so a compromise is reached between acceptable tissue damage and efficiency of grip. This compromise will alter from case to case. Thin-walled, floppy gallbladders are most easily damaged and are best gripped with atraumatic forceps. Thick-walled inflamed gallbladders slip out of atraumatic forceps and toothed or 'claw' forceps may be required. Heavy duty 10 mm grasping forceps are used to draw the gallbladder into the cannula prior to its removal.

Stone removal forceps

These are 10 mm instruments with cupped jaws which can be used to scoop up loose stones.

Needle holders

A laparoscopic needle holder must grip the needle securely preventing rotation, be easy to rotate in one's palm when suturing, and able to release the needle smoothly without jerking.

A spring-handled atraumatic grasping/dissecting forceps will hold a needle, but allows it to rotate within the jaws. An alternative is the Cook needle holder (Fig. 2.6), in which a central oblique piston closes on the needle to hold it firmly in position, preventing rotation.

Conventional handles are better replaced by a cylindrical handle

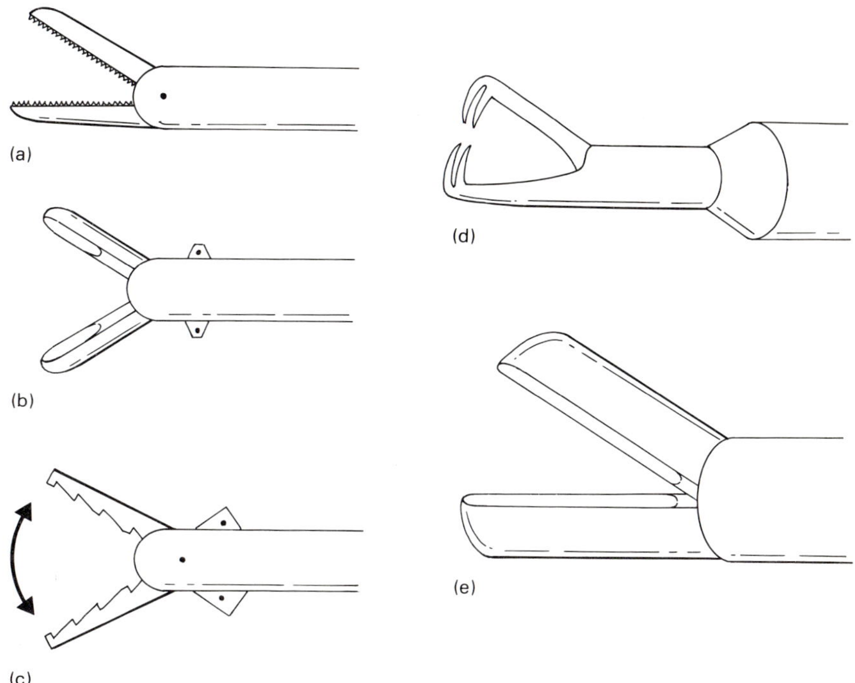

Fig. 2.5 Different types of jaws for grasping forceps.

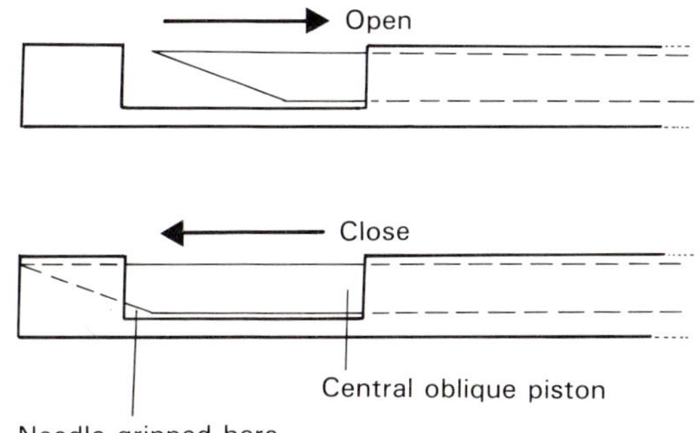

Fig. 2.6 The Cook needle holder: one design of needle holder.

which sits in one's palm and which can be easily rotated in the palm, with a trigger to release the needle.

Dissecting instruments

Specialized dissecting instruments such as the Petelin forceps are modifications of the grasping/holding forceps, facilitating blunt dissection especially around Calot's triangle. A curved, atraumatic forceps allows easy isolation of duct and artery with minimal damage. Whether insulated or not, these dissecting instruments should have a matt black finish to eliminate reflected glare back to the laparoscope.

Suction/irrigation devices

In order to keep a clear view of the operative field, a variety of suction/irrigation devices have been developed. Irrigating fluid

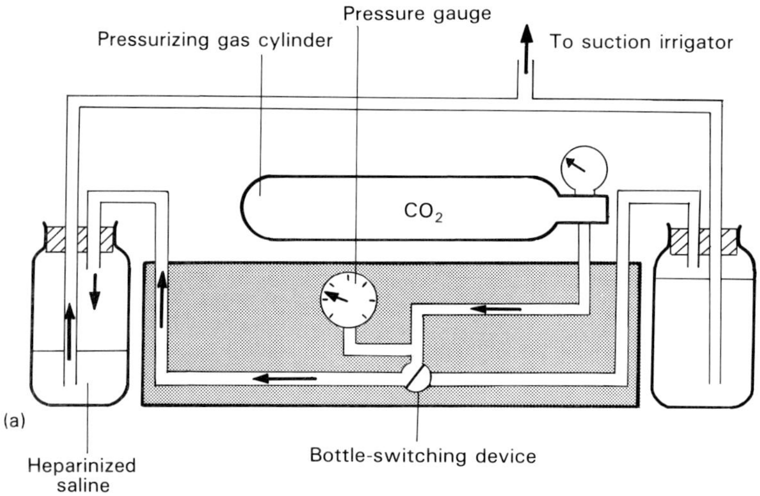

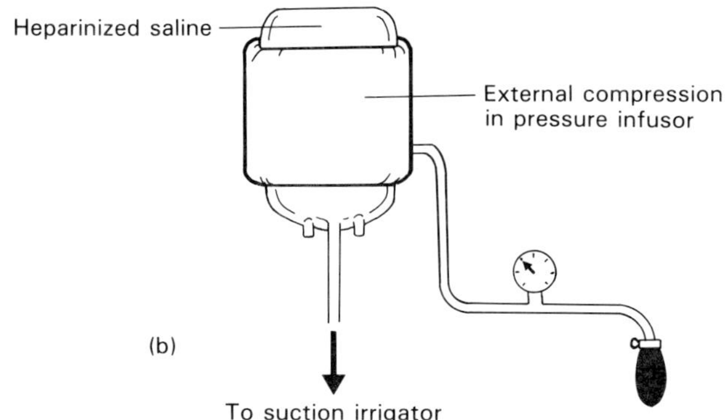

Fig. 2.7 Schematic diagram of suction and irrigation apparatus. An alternative is a pressurized intravenous saline bag.

(heparinized saline) is delivered under pressure to wash away blood clots and loose tissue debris. It also allows the identification of particular bleeding points prior to cautery. The fluid is delivered under pressure (400–500 mmHg). This pressure can be achieved either by external compression of a saline bag in a pressure-infusor similar to that used for rapid blood transfusion, or by pressurizing a bottle of saline with CO_2 (Fig. 2.7).

The addition of heparin to the irrigating saline (1000 units per litre) is made to prevent blood collecting and forming large clots which are then difficult to aspirate.

The ideal suction/irrigation device combines both in one probe, with the flow controlled by either a tap or trumpet valve. One such device, the Nehzat probe, is illustrated in Fig. 2.8. Some single channel probes are insulated to their tip to permit cautery and either irrigation or aspiration. The authors do not find this as convenient as having both suction and irrigation combined in the same instrument.

Notes

1 When using irrigating saline pressurized by CO_2 care should be taken when the saline runs out, since CO_2 will then be pumped through the irrigating probe under pressure and cause a rapid rise in intra-abdominal pressure.

2 Inadvertent suction, or prolonged suction will remove CO_2 from the abdomen causing rapid loss of pneumoperitoneum.

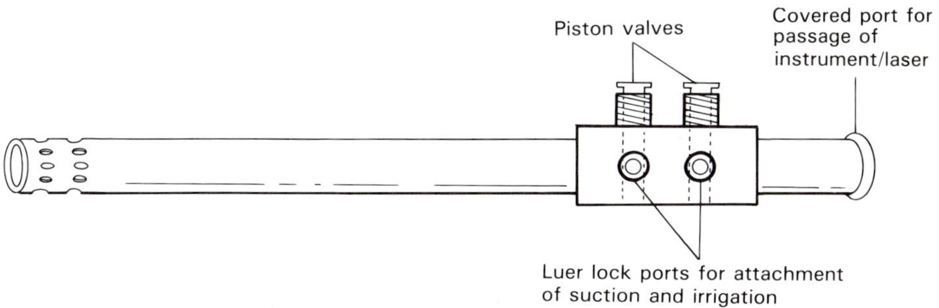

Fig. 2.8 The Nehzat probe allows both suction and irrigation. These functions are controlled by separate piston valves. A small instrument such as a laser fibre can pass down the central channel.

Sutures

In order to pass down a trocar laparoscopic sutures are limited in design. Currently available sutures have a 'ski needle', shaped like a ski in profile (Fig. 2.9), with a round body on cross-section. The suture material, commonly polyglactin (Vicryl, Ethicon Ltd) is swaged onto the needle and is shorter in length than normal sutures to facilitate tying.

Notes

The suture should be introduced via a 10 mm cannula, with a 5 mm forceps/needle holder holding the thread and leading the needle down behind. Once inside the needle can be picked up. A similar thread first technique is required for removal.

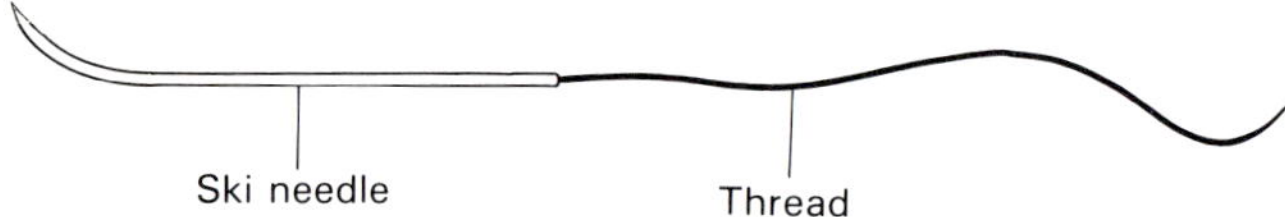

Fig. 2.9 The type of needle used in laparoscopic surgery has to be able to go through the laparoscopic cannula.

Clip appliers

The application of a small clip is adequate to completely occlude both cystic artery and cystic duct, and thus obviates the need to ligate either of these structures during laparoscopic cholecystectomy. Two types of clip are available, one metal the other manufactured from Polydioxanone (PDS) (Ligaclip and Absolok, respectively, manufactured by Ethicon Ltd).

The metal clip appliers are 10 mm instruments which introduce the clip into the abdomen in the open position. The jaws are placed around the vessel or duct to be occluded and brought together by squeezing the instrument's handles, thus crushing the clip. When the clip is crushed, the tips of the clip are brought together first before the body of the clip is closed (Fig. 2.10). It is important not to have any tissue trapped beyond the jaws of the clip applier or else it is unable to occlude the vessel/duct securely. The clips themselves are either 6 or 9 mm in length.

Clip appliers come either as single reusable instruments which are reloaded after each application, or multiple clip applicators which

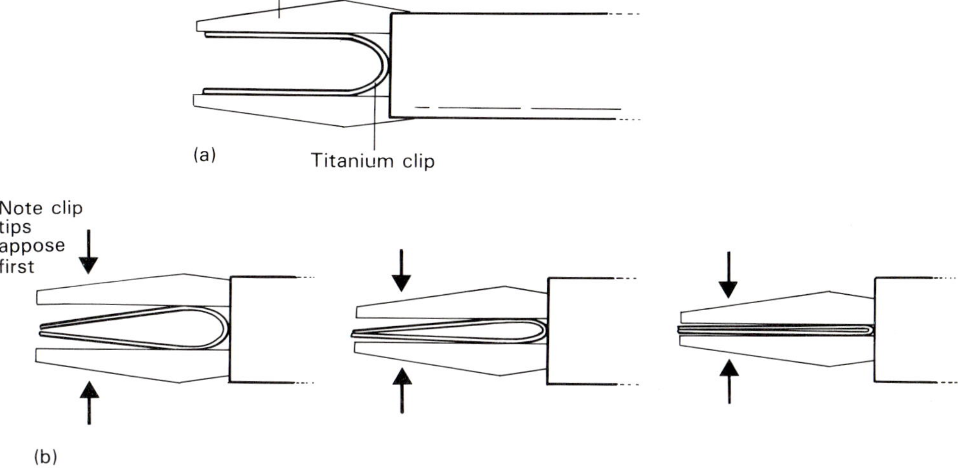

Fig. 2.10 Clip applicators close the tips of the clip first.

have 10–15 clips and are capable of sequential firing while remaining in the abdomen.

Absolok clips work differently. They rely on their tips interlocking beyond the vessel/duct to be occluded (see Fig. 4.16). Hence it is just as important when applying these clips to 'clean' the vessel to allow the clip to engage without any tissue obstructing the clip mechanism.

Notes

1 It is important to ensure that the clips pass across the vessel/duct to be occluded to ensure safe application. If this is not possible a ligature should be used.

2 Single reusable metal clip appliers are adequate for normal gallbladder operations. However, multiple clip appliers are useful where difficulties such as bleeding vessels are encountered.

3 The novice will find it difficult to reintroduce the instrument to the same position after reloading. This is made easier if the assistant holds the cannula fixed in the same orientation while the instrument is removed for reloading.

4 For added safety at least two clips should be applied on the patient side of any major vessel or duct to be divided.

5 Metal clips are likely to interfere with magnetic resonance imaging.

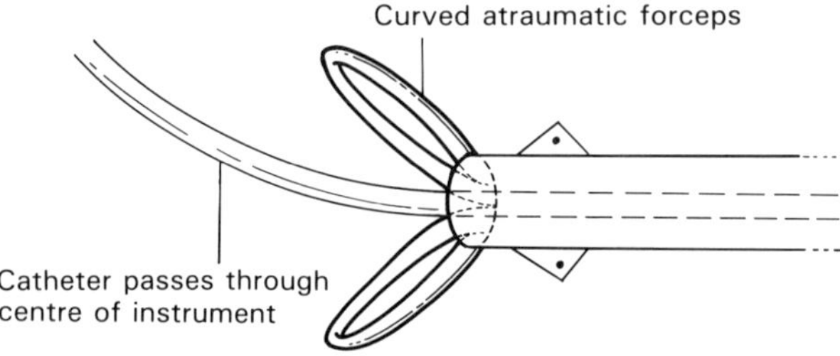

Fig. 2.11 The Reddick–Olsen cholangiogram clamp. Once the catheter is in the cystic duct it and the duct are grasped by the atraumatic jaws.

Specialized instruments

Reddick–Olsen cholangiography clamp (Fig. 2.11)

The cholangiography clamp is an atraumatic double-hinged grasping forceps with curved jaws, a central lumen through the shaft and a ratchet on the handles. Through the central lumen a small catheter is passed and directed through an incision in the cystic duct. The jaws are then closed holding the duct around the cannula. This instrument is then left in place while the cholangiogram is performed.

Notes
1 The instrument should be used through the subcostal port, so that it does not overlie the common bile duct.
2 The patency of the central lumen should be checked before use.

Cholangiography catheter

We use a cannula/catheter set used for jugular or subclavian vein cannulation (Wallace piggy back central venous catheter). This comprises a small 16 gauge catheter and needle and a larger 13 gauge cannula. The 13 gauge cannula and the needle are pushed through the abdominal wall and the needle removed. The 16 gauge catheter is then passed through the lumen of the cannula into the abdomen.

Dormia basket

Designed primarily for urological use, the Dormia basket removes stones from the bile duct with equal facility as from the ureter. It is made up of four wires which retract into a sheath (we use a 4.5

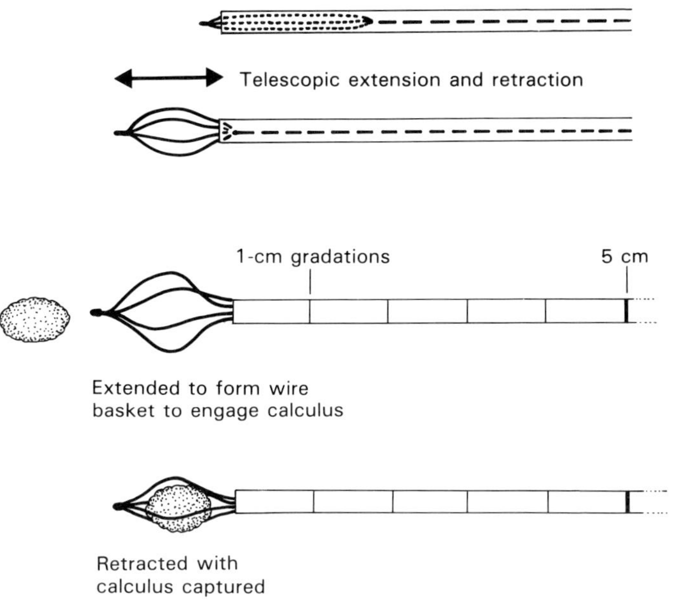

Fig. 2.12 The Dormia basket. The wire basket is extruded in order to trap a stone. The stone is held when the basket is retracted.

French gauge basket). When extended, the wires form a basket into which stones can be trapped (Fig. 2.12). When retracted the basket and the stone are withdrawn from the duct. The outer cannula cover is marked at 1 and 5 cm intervals.

Notes
1 Do not be afraid to use several baskets for multiple stones. After several attempts to capture stones, successful or otherwise, the Dormia basket function becomes impaired, particularly if the wires have been bent and remodelled.
2 Be gentle. The basket can trap biliary epithelium if used repeatedly especially if the basket itself has been bent. Damage to biliary epithelium may lead to bleeding, oedema and stricture.

3: Lasers and laparoscopic surgery

What is a laser?
  Production of laser energy
  Properties of laser light
  Pulsed and continuous-wave mode
    lasers

Laser–tissue interactions
Dangers of lasers
  Characteristics of different lasers
Delivery of laser light
Contact lasers

What is a laser?

A laser is amplified light of very high energy. It is produced by energizing the atoms in a 'lasing medium'. Each atom consists of a central nucleus and its orbiting electrons. The electrons orbit at predefined distances from the nucleus, the basic orbit being known as the ground state. If external energy is introduced, electrons may be raised to a higher orbit (excited) by the addition of a defined package or quantum of energy (Fig. 3.1).

Once excited, the electron remains in that state for a very brief period before regaining equilibrium by returning to its normal orbit. As it falls back into its normal orbit, the energy initially absorbed is released as a photon. The photon has a wavelength characteristic to that particular medium (Fig. 3.2).

Having been released, the photon travels on to strike another atom which may also be in an excited state. As this electron returns to equilibrium, two identical photons are emitted (Fig. 3.3).

When this process takes place in a confined space with parallel mirrors at each end (resonator), the number of photons released rises on a massive scale. Photons are reflected backwards and forwards

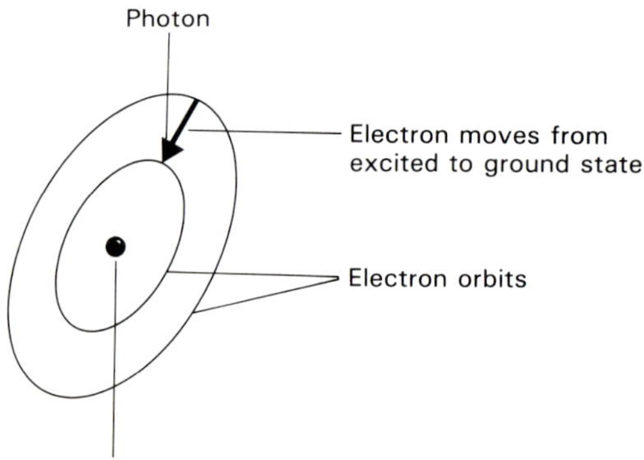

Fig. 3.1 An excited electron emits a photon when returning to its resting orbit.

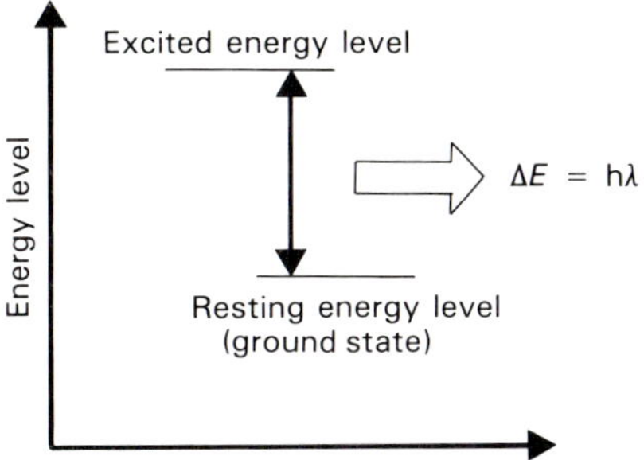

Fig. 3.2 The energy released is related to the frequency of the light emitted.

between the mirrors and establish a pattern of parallel high energy light. Once the number of excited atoms outnumbers the atoms in the resting state a condition known as 'population inversion' occurs producing amplification of light. If one of the mirrors is 90% reflective, 10% of the high energy light within the chamber can be released. The result is Light Amplification by the Stimulated Emission of Radiation, or a LASER beam.

Production of laser energy
In order to generate laser light, energy is applied to a 'lasing' medium to raise its atoms from their ground state to an excited level. The medium is activated in a resonator by an energy source called the excitation pump. The energy source may take many forms, such as

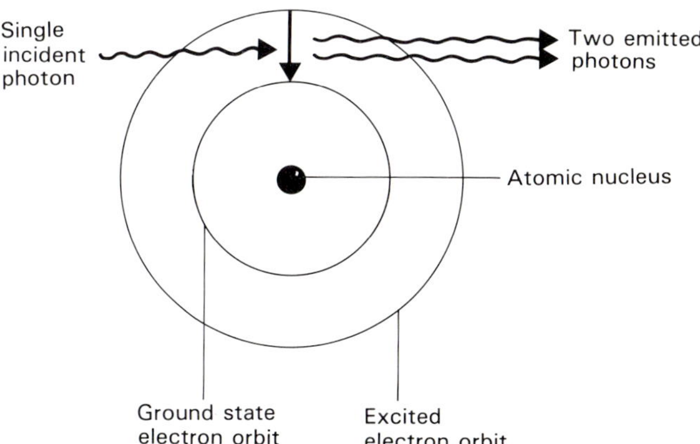

Fig. 3.3 Photon stimulating emission of identical photon. When a photon strikes an electron which is already in an excited state, two identical photons are emitted.

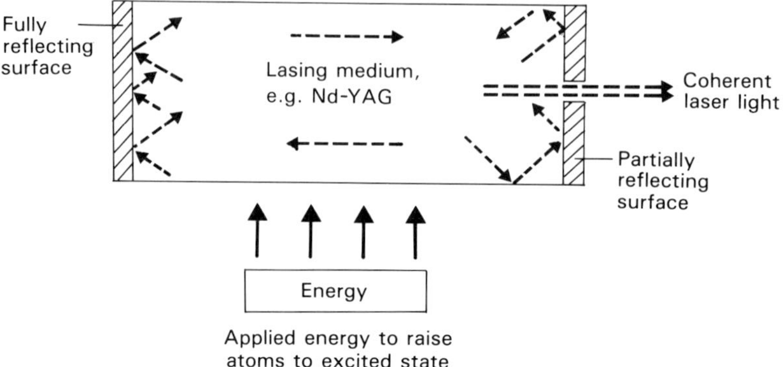

Fig. 3.4 Schematic diagram of a laser resonator.

a flash light, an electrical discharge, or another laser (Fig. 3.4). The reflected light within the chamber stimulates further laser energy production from the lasing medium.

Properties of laser light
1 Monochromatic. The laser light comprises photons of identical wavelength, or colour.
2 Collimated. The light waves are parallel, neither diverging nor converging.
3 Coherent. The light waves are equal and in phase.

Pulsed and continuous-wave mode lasers
Laser energy can be continuously delivered (continuous-wave) or released in short pulses of less than 0.25 second duration (pulsed). Pulsed lasers deliver short bursts of high power, while continuous-wave mode delivers a constant power level. In laparoscopic surgical practice the constant power level afforded in the continuous-wave mode is preferable.

Laser–tissue interactions
When a laser beam comes into contact with a surface one of four things may happen.
1 Reflection.
2 Scattering.
3 Transmission.
4 Absorption.

Which of these occurs depends upon the characteristics of the laser light itself as well as on the nature and colour of the incident surface.

Dangers of lasers

As long as the laser beam remains coherent and collimated it can damage structures in its path. As the laser light can be reflected off shiny surfaces the use of a laser beam carries considerable potential for accidental damage away from the operation site. The beam can be reflected onto other structures, can burn structures beyond the tissue being divided ('past burning'), and can be reflected back up optical fibres to damage the eye of the operator. A laser beam striking the macula will produce permanent blindness.

Because of these dangers the law requires everyone in the operating theatre to wear suitable protective glasses and to take various other precautions. The laser company will inform you of these.

The dangers can be considerably diminished by avoiding the use of bare fibre lasers and focusing the beam with a contact tip (see below). As the beam loses its power beyond the contact tip, the only remaining dangers are due to accidental breakage of the transmitting fibre.

Characteristics of different lasers

The characteristics of the atoms comprising the 'lasing' medium dictate the frequency (and therefore wavelength) of the laser light, since the energy released by the atom as its electron moves from the excited state to the ground state is directly proportional to the frequency of the emitted light radiation.

Carbon dioxide (CO_2) lasers

Carbon dioxide (CO_2) lasers emit light of frequency 10 590 nm (in the far infrared end of the spectrum). Because of their long wavelength they cannot be delivered via an optical fibre. Instead they require an articulated arm with mirrors at each articulation to direct the laser beam in the required direction. Since the beam is invisible it requires a second, visible, aiming beam, typically a low power helium–neon (He–Ne) laser. The CO_2 laser beam is well absorbed by water and since most tissue is more than 80% water, virtually all CO_2 energy is absorbed within 0.2 mm of the tissue surface. This makes the CO_2

laser a good cutting instrument producing a sharp incision with minimal lateral necrosis. The CO_2 beam must be focused onto the treatment site. It is used principally in gynaecology for the treatment of premalignant cervical lesions.

The argon laser

Argon laser energy is characterized by two peaks, at wavelengths of 488 and 514 nm (blue and blue–green end of visible spectrum respectively). A laser beam of this wavelength will pass through water and clear media (such as the vitreous of the eye) with very little effect; it reacts with red tissue and is primarily absorbed by tissue pigments such as haemoglobin and melanin. It has a tissue penetration of about 1 mm and will coagulate small vessels but not large ones. Argon lasers are large and have an efficiency of 0.01% compared to the 20% efficiency of a CO_2 laser. Their ability to pass through the humours of the eye has led to their widespread use in ophthalmology.

The KTP laser

This uses potassium (K^+) titanyl (T) phosphate (P) which emits green light with a wavelength of 532 nm. The energy source may be a YAG laser (see below). The beam is suitable for cutting or coagulation and a bare fibre is used. Placed in contact with tissues (without a tip) the laser has good cutting characteristics. When used away from the tissues the defocused beam produces coagulation. As it is a bare fibre laser, past burning and reflection have to be guarded against.

The Nd–YAG laser

The laser medium is yttrium aluminium garnet (YAG), a crystal which is used in artificial diamonds. This has incorporated into it a trace quantity of the rare earth neodymium (Nd) which serves as the actual lasing medium. The wavelength produced, 1060 nm, is in the near infrared region of the spectrum. The beam is invisible and an additional He–Ne aiming beam is required, as with the CO_2 laser. Because of its relatively short wavelength, unlike the CO_2 laser, the Nd–YAG laser beam can be transmitted through optical fibres and hence delivered through all flexible fibreoptic endoscopes. It passes through water with little effect and can therefore be used in the bladder and other fluid-filled cavities. It passes through tissue and penetrates to a depth of 5 mm. It is absorbed by tissue proteins and delivers a broad non-specific thermal effect which makes it an excellent coagulator even at sites of active bleeding. The main problem with the Nd–YAG laser is that the light is scattered when it strikes a tissue and thus loses much of its energy. The beam tends to do more damage to adjacent healthy tissue than the CO_2 laser. Nd–YAG lasers are extremely reliable and easy to maintain.

Delivery of laser light

A CO_2 laser has to be delivered down an articulated arm system containing mirrors.

Lasers of shorter wavelengths such as the Nd–YAG can be transmitted down flexible fibres. One problem with such fibre delivery system is that the beam tends to diverge as it emerges from the end of the fibre. Once it diverges, the concentration of energy (spot size) is widened and it loses its power.

Contact lasers

One way to get around the problem of divergence at the end of a fibre is to fix a conical sapphire tip to the end of the fibre. This focuses the beam at the tip of the crystal and this has many beneficial effects.

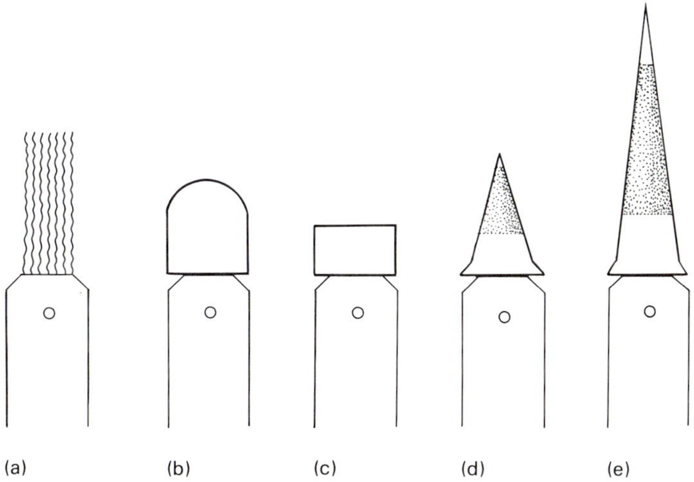

Fig. 3.5 Different contact tip laser probes produce different tissue interactions. (a) Bare laser fibre; (b) round probe (vaporization); (c) flat probe (coagulation); (d, e) scalpel probe (point for cutting, frosted side for coagulation).

1 As the energy is focused and the spot size diminished, less power (watts) is required to generate a similar tissue effect.

2 As the energy is only concentrated on the tip of the crystal, there are no effects beyond the tip and distant burns and reflection of laser light are not a problem.

3 As the laser is used in contact with the tissue, tactile sensation (similar to using a scalpel) is reintroduced giving the surgeon greater feedback and control.

Different types of tips can be fitted to a laser fibre giving different characteristics (Fig. 3.5).

Disadvantages of contact tip lasers included the need to change these tips for different functions, and that the tips are expensive and need regular replacement.

4: Laparoscopic techniques

Converting to laparoscopic
    operative techniques
Producing a pneumoperitoneum
  Safety tests
Initial laparoscopy
Retraction
Inserting an extra port
Dissection/haemostasis
  Using the diathermy hook
  Dissecting scissors
  Using the laser

Blunt dissection
Suction and irrigation
Clips
  Multifire clip applicator
  Self-locking clips
Tying knots and suturing
  External knotting (Roeder knot)
  Preformed catgut ligatures
  Suturing
  Internal knots

Converting to laparoscopic operative techniques

Operating and using a laparoscope is initially difficult due to the need to operate by 'remote control' with a two-dimensional image produced by a camera, instead of normal stereoscopic direct vision. This problem can be greatly increased if the image is not correctly orientated or the operating ports are incorrectly sited. Ideally the surgeon's head should be on a line with the camera and the laparoscope, and the screen visible along the same line (see Fig. 4.3). The camera image should also remain correctly orientated in space, i.e. the camera and laparoscope must not be rotated (Fig. 4.1). If a rotation of 90° clockwise does occur, for instance, an instrument entering the abdomen at 45° from the vertical (Fig. 4.2) on the right side will appear on the screen to enter from 135°. The camera person should have this phenomenon demonstrated at the beginning of the operation. The surgeon will quickly become sensitive to this cause of disorientation.

It is also important to position the 'left hand' and 'right hand' ports forward and lateral to the camera port (Fig. 4.3). Ideally all three should be at the points of an equilateral triangle and meet at the operative site slightly ahead of the instrument holding ports. If these ports are too close to the laparoscope, the instruments in them will interfere with vision. If they are too far forward the operator will be working with the instrument pointing towards the camera and movements will be reversed.

During the operation the non-dominant (usually the left) hand is more important than in open surgery. In laparoscopic surgery the movements of the right hand are severely restricted by the fixed position of the operative port. The left hand has therefore to move

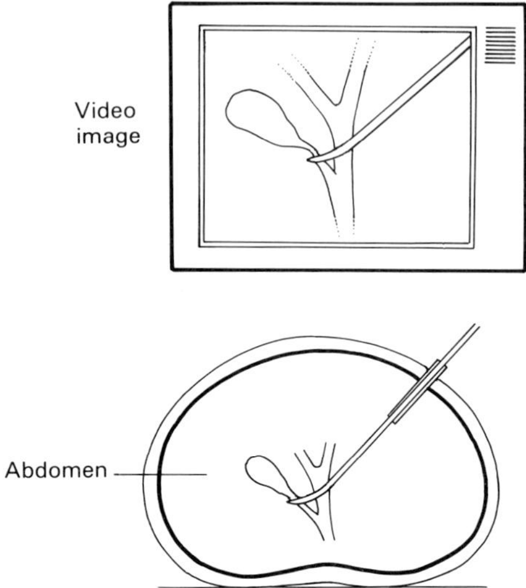

Fig. 4.1 With the camera held straight the image on the video screen is in the same orientation as the situation in the abdomen.

structures to an optimal position where the instrument in the right hand can get at them. It also has to frequently change grip and tension on the structure held, in order to aid dissection.

Many apparent difficulties can be solved by paying attention to the position maintained by the grasper in the left hand.

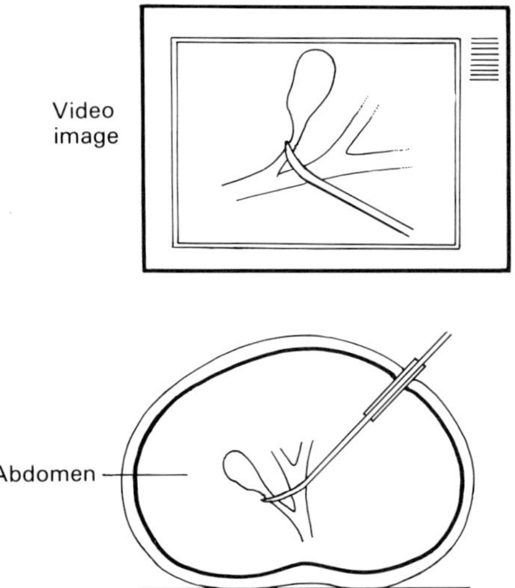

Fig. 4.2 When the camera is rotated 90° the video image is no longer correctly related to the situation in the abdomen.

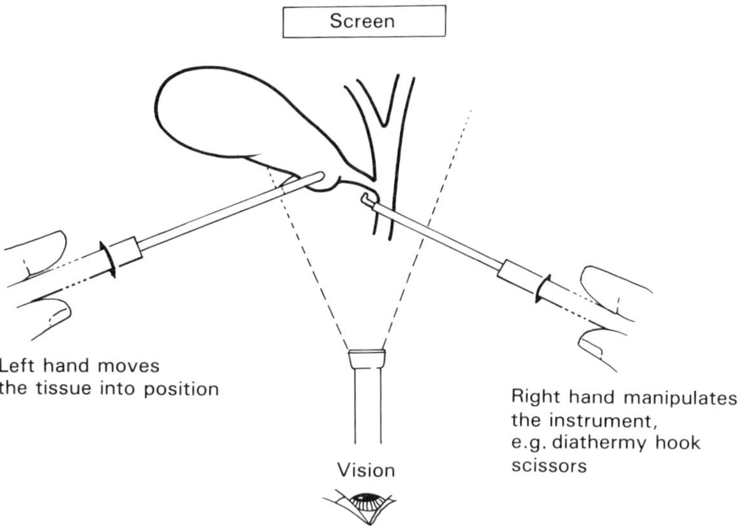

Fig. 4.3 Hand/eye coordination is easiest if the surgeon's eye, laparoscope, and the screen are in a direct line. The left hand and right hand instrument ports should be in front of and lateral to the laparoscope port.

Finally, the lack of stereoscopic vision can be overcome by 'fixing' the position of a structure by moving an instrument first in front and then behind it (Fig. 4.4). This 'fore and aft' technique is particularly useful when cutting sutures or opening the cystic duct.

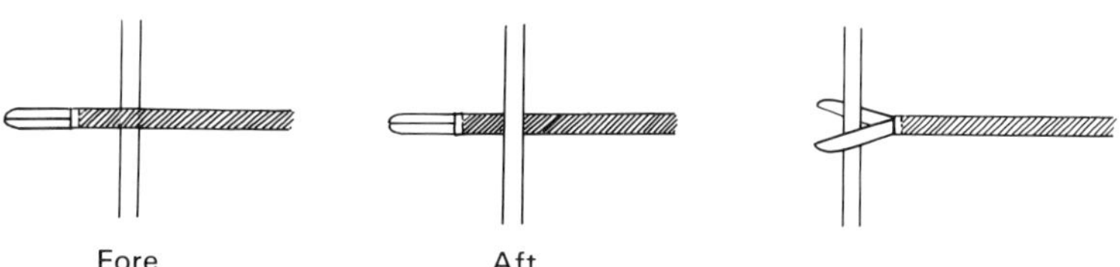

Fig. 4.4 The fore and aft technique: the position of a structure in space can be determined by passing an instrument before and behind it.

Producing a pneumoperitoneum

Technique

A Verres needle is inserted into the peritoneal space and CO_2 insufflated, thus separating the anterior abdominal wall from the peritoneal contents (Fig. 4.5).

Hold the Verres needle by the moveable outer sheath so that the

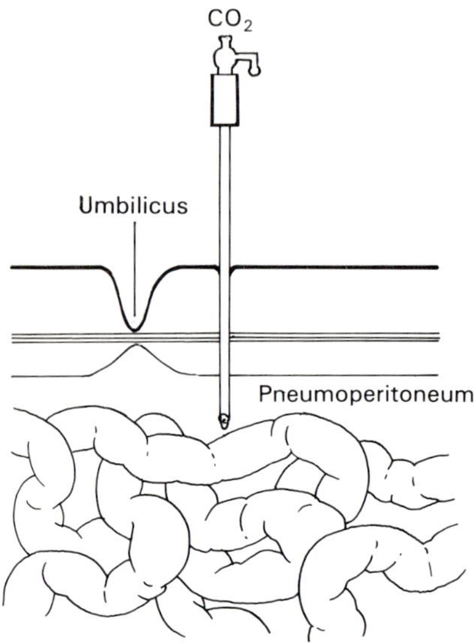

Fig. 4.5 Inducing a pneumoperitoneum with the Verres needle.

blunt trocar is free to retract and spring forward, not by the outer fixed end.

An initial incision is made either just below, just above, or through the umbilical scar. The incision measures about 2 cm across, just large enough to take the 10 mm cannula. We use a supra-umbilical incision routinely.

Grasp the full thickness of the abdominal wall in your left hand, either below the umbilicus or, with an assistant, on both sides of the umbilicus. This provides counter-traction against the needle and allows the bowel to fall away as soon as gas is introduced.

Holding the needle between your thumb and forefinger like a dart, pull up the skin and muscle and aim the needle for the pelvic cavity at an angle of 45° down towards the feet, carefully pushing it through the abdominal wall. A definite give is usually experienced when it passes through the peritoneum into the peritoneal cavity.

At this point safety tests are carried out to confirm that the needle is truly in the peritoneal cavity.

Safety tests

1 Vacuum test. A drop of saline is placed on the open end of the Verres needle. Lifting up the abdominal wall will create a negative pressure in the peritoneal cavity and the saline drop is sucked down.

2 Syringe test. A syringe is attached to the luer lock of the Verres

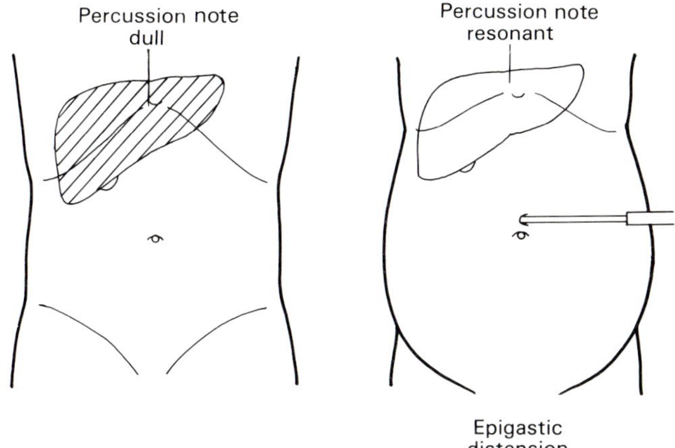

Fig. 4.6 With gas in the peritoneum the liver dullness disappears and the epigastrium becomes distended.

needle, and 10 ml of saline injected. If the needle is in the peritoneal cavity the saline flows away easily, and none can be aspirated back. If fluid is aspirated back, the needle is probably extraperitoneal and needs repositioning. Aspiration of blood or bowel contents also indicates incorrect needle placement.

3 Free movement test. Check that the tip of the needle moves freely from side to side. Undue resistance to movement may indicate that it has penetrated a peritoneal structure or posterior wall.

Initial insufflation is carried out at a low rate of flow (1 litre per minute). The insufflator should indicate that gas is flowing freely and the insufflation pressure should remain low (less than 10 mmHg). If that is not the case, resite the needle since the needle is either still in the abdominal wall or is against a viscus.

It is helpful to have noted the needle's own resistance to gas flow by observing pressures at low and high gas flow rates before the needle is inserted.

Percuss over the liver to check that the dullness is disappearing (Fig. 4.6). This occurs after about 500 ml of CO_2. Once you are sure that the insufflation gas is in the right place, increase the flow to 4 litres per minute until the abdomen is satisfactorily distended or approximately 3 litres of CO_2 have been instilled. The intraperitoneal pressure is maintained at 10–15 mmHg when adequately distended.

Dangers
1 Surgical emphysema. Surgical emphysema due to CO_2 is not a serious condition and will rapidly be absorbed. If the Verres needle is in the subcutaneous or extraperitoneal tissues, surgical emphysema will be produced with a characteristic subcutaneous crackling feel. Cease insufflation immediately and reposition the needle. In extreme cases the subcutaneous tissues of the genitalia or head, neck and face may be affected.
2 CO_2 embolism (see also Chapter 6, p. 64). If the needle penetrates a vessel there is a danger of CO_2 embolism. The anaesthetist will spot a sudden fall in end-tidal CO_2 (due to lack of perfusion of lung capillaries), and circulatory collapse may follow. Cease insufflating immediately and desufflate the abdomen. Tilt the table foot up.
3 Perforation of the bowel or other viscera (see Chapter 9, p. 121).
4 Penetration of major posterior retroperitoneal vessels such as the aorta or inferior vena cava (see Chapter 9, p. 113).

Hints
Use a guarded (e.g. Verres) needle for creation of the pneumo-peritoneum.

Initial laparoscopy

This can be carried out once the second port is in place or delayed until all four ports have been inserted.

Technique
At initial laparoscopy, look around the peritoneal cavity and note the presence and site of adhesions. This will define areas that cannot be easily visualized and a decision may be made whether it is necessary to divide any adhesions before further laparoscopic surgery can be undertaken.

Look for blood in the loops of bowel beneath the port sites particularly underneath the initial (umbilical) site. If there is bleeding it will usually stop quite quickly. Otherwise proceed as in Chapter 9, p. 112. Check there is no retroperitoneal haematoma.

Look down towards the pelvis and inspect the pelvic organs. The graspers in port 2 or port 3 can be used to manipulate the pelvic organs or occasionally the blunt tip of a Verres needle inserted independently in the iliac fossa can be of value.

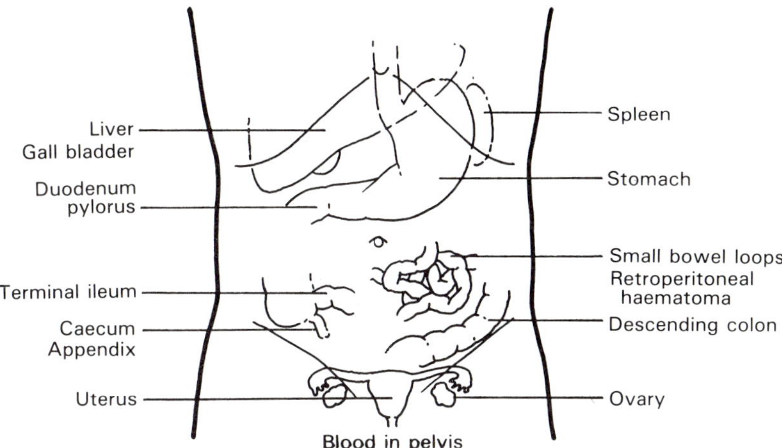

Fig. 4.7 A routine laparoscopy inspection of the abdominal organs should always be carried out.

Move around to the left and inspect the descending colon, spleen, stomach and hiatus (Fig. 4.7).

Withdraw the laparoscope slightly to pass underneath the falciform ligament and inspect the rest of the liver, the right upper quadrant and finally the gallbladder.

Retraction

Abdominal wall

As in other forms of surgery good retraction is essential in order to achieve a satisfactory view. Unlike open surgery however, there is no need to retract the abdominal wall as this is held away by the pneumoperitoneum.

Gallbladder

Retraction of the gallbladder is dealt with on p. 85.

Falciform lift

The falciform lift is a technique to retract the falciform ligament, and with it the left hepatic lobe, upwards. It is seldom necessary if the epigastric cannula (port 4) is introduced to the right of the falciform ligament on initial entry.

Technique

A heavy prolene suture (1/0) on a long straight cutting needle is pushed vertically through the skin and into the peritoneal cavity to the left of the midline under direct vision. Once inside, it is seized by forceps, passed beneath and to the right of the falciform ligament, before being pushed back out of the peritoneal cavity. Once outside, the two ends may either be tied or beads crushed to hold them in place, pulling the ligamentum teres and falciform ligament upwards against the abdominal wall. The more cranial the suture is placed, the better the retraction.

Dangers
1 Puncture of epigastric vessels.
2 Puncture of viscera.

Hints
1 Identify large vessels by illuminating the abdominal wall from below with the laparoscope before puncture.
2 Always introduce the needle under direct vision.

Inserting an extra port

Technique
Occasionally it is necessary to insert an extra port to push the colon or omentum out of the way. This may be avoided if a 25/30° scope is available (see p. 111). The extra port can be inserted in the right lower abdomen, lateral to port 3, and a grasper used to pull the colon down. A subcostal port with a grasper pushing the colon downwards is also a possibility though this tends to obstruct the operating ports.

Dissection/haemostasis

As in open surgery, laparoscopic dissection is a combination of blunt dissection, sharp dissection and haemostasis. In order to minimize instrument changes many laparoscopic instruments are insulated to permit them to be used for electrocautery as well as for their prime function.

Using the diathermy hook
This is extremely useful both for dissection and haemostasis.

Technique
When dissecting the peritoneum off the cystic duct or Calot's triangle,

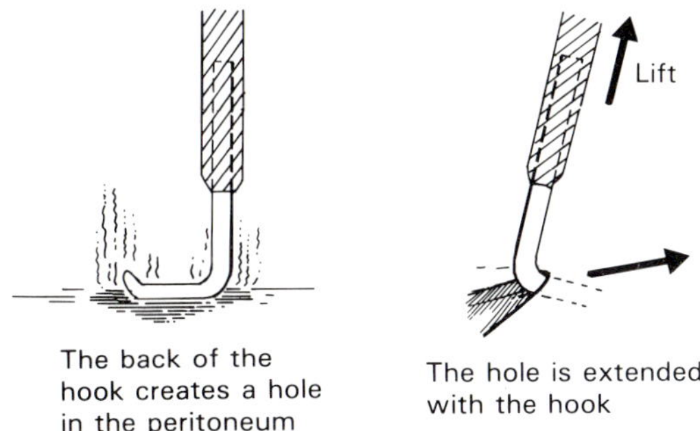

Fig. 4.8 Use of the hook diathermy to create a hole in, and then to divide, the peritoneum.

an initial small burn can be made by touching the peritoneum with the back of the hook. The point of the hook can then be inserted and the peritoneum lifted away from the underlying structures (Fig. 4.8). Further diathermy will then continue to divide the peritoneum.

The hook is also useful for dividing strands of tissue around the cystic duct and attached to the gallbladder. Hook the instrument under the strand of tissue (hook), apply traction to keep the metal away from neighbouring structures, and check that the hooked structure is suitable for division (look). Once you are sure it is safe, press the pedal and divide the strand by diathermy (cook) (Fig. 4.9). Alternatively, the back of the hook can be used to divide tissues, or separate the gallbladder from its bed, provided that good retraction places the tissue to be divided on the stretch.

Dangers
It is easy to cause a deep burn and partially damage a larger vessel situated deeply. There are particular dangers while dissecting in

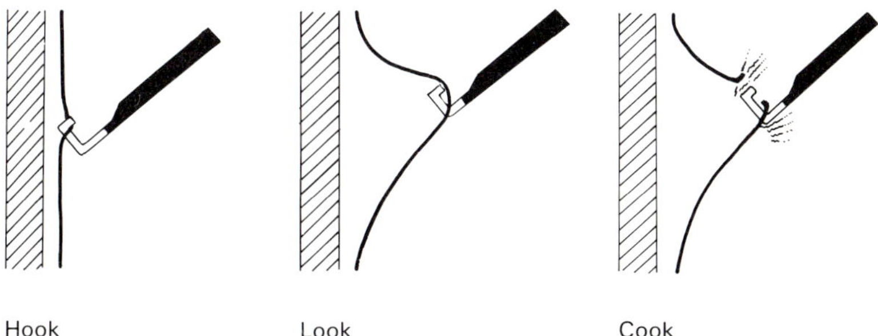

Fig. 4.9 Diathermy hook. Always retract a strand away from the underlying structures and inspect it before applying the diathermy current.

Calot's triangle close to the right lobe of the liver over the right hepatic duct and right branch of the portal vein. The heat from the diathermy spreads for at least 5 mm and more if pedal pressure is continued.

After prolonged diathermy, the tip of the hook remains hot and can easily burn a hole in a neighbouring viscus.

The wall of a large vessel damaged by diathermy may not give way until a few days after the operation. When the slough separates, the patient suffers an unexpected bleed.

Hints
Use the routine of hook, look, cook to ensure safety. Do not diathermy too much tissue at once. Use repeated small burns. Allow the tip to cool after use before allowing it to lie on any intra-abdominal structures; dipping the tip in the pool of peritoneal fluid hastens cooling.

Dissecting scissors

Technique
Put the tissue on the stretch by retracting the gallbladder with the graspers in your left hand. Cut the visible stretched tissue, cauterizing with the scissors first if necessary.

Dangers
Do not conduct the diathermy heat through the sharp edge of the scissors as this will help to blunt them.

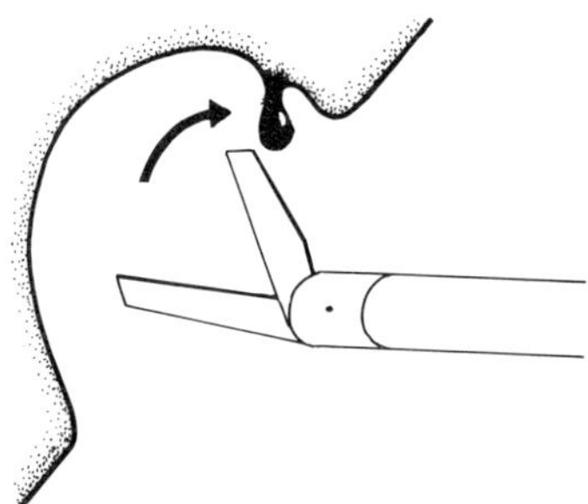

Fig. 4.10 The back of the open scissors can be used to diathermy round a corner.

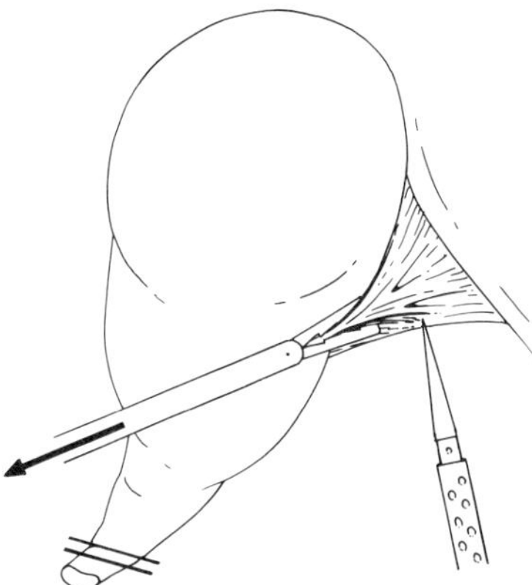

Fig. 4.11 Tissue should be put on the stretch before dividing it with a contact tip laser (scalpel tip).

Hints
Diathermy with the back of the scissors. Using the scissors open it is possible to diathermy around a corner with the back of the blade (Fig. 4.10).

Using the laser
The theory behind the use of the laser is given in Chapter 3.

Technique
It is essential to stretch the tissue to be divided before applying the laser (Fig. 4.11).

When using a bare fibre laser it is important to take note of what is on the far side of the tissue you are going to divide. This will also be damaged once the laser cuts through the target tissue.

Dangers of bare fibre
1 Burns of distant tissue.
2 Penetration of other organs.
3 Perforation of the diaphragm.

Contact tip laser (Figs 4.12, 4.13)
Touch the tissue to be divided using a sweeping motion of the sapphire tip. If the vessels are present, coagulate them with the side of the contact tip before dividing them.

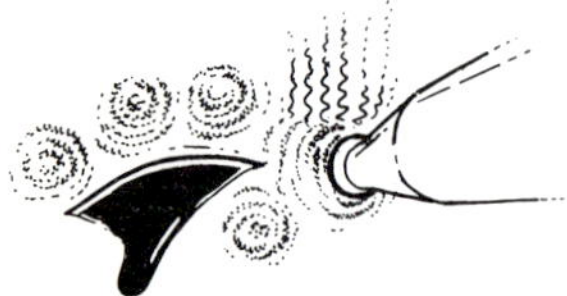

Fig. 4.12 The coagulating contact tip can be used to create a rosette around a bleeding vessel. A bare fibre laser can also be used for this purpose.

Dangers of contact tip

1 This is very 'sharp'. It is easy to penetrate the gallblader or the liver and it is essential to line up the tissues to be divided accurately before pressing the foot pedal.

2 If the tip is inserted deep into the liver there is a danger of embolism from the CO_2 gas used to cool the laser tip.

3 If the sapphire contact tip is heated up for prolonged periods when it is not in contact with tissue it will burn out.

Hints

With a contact tip laser, fire the laser for a second or so before touching any tissue. This warms up the tip which then cuts immediately in contact with tissue.

Manoeuvre the tissue with the left hand to place it where you can reach it with the laser at the correct angle.

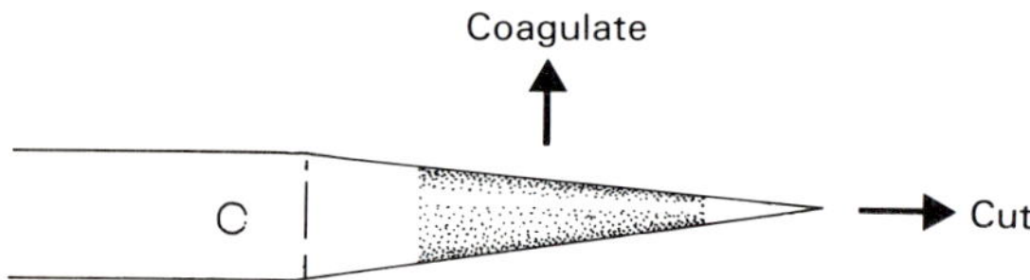

Fig. 4.13 A frosted contact laser tip produces coagulation from the side and cutting at the tip.

Blunt dissection

A variety of instruments can be used to tease or tear structures apart. There are several specially designed instruments but both the scissors and the diathermy hook can be used for this purpose. The special instruments may either have straight jaws or curved (e.g. Petelin's forceps), and one or both jaws may open.

Technique

Pick up the strand and pull it gently, separating it from its attachments. Find the layer between two structures and gently open and close the jaws of the instruments to separate them.

Dangers
If the bands are strong this technique may result in perforation or shredding of the gallbladder, cystic duct, common bile duct or vessels.

Hints
Always keep the plane of dissection close to the viscus wall. Dissect close to the gallbladder, away from the common bile duct.

Suction and irrigation
Suction and irrigation instruments are described in Chapter 2.

Technique
Wash the desired area with a low flow of heparinized saline. Retrieve the fluid by sucking in the fossa either between the liver and duodenum or lateral to the liver.

Dangers
1 If too high a pressure is used, the saline may splash onto the camera obscuring the view. This is particularly troublesome when the camera is very close to the dissection.
2 Suction above the level of fluid empties the pneumoperitoneum.
3 Stones may block the sucker or cause the trumpet valve to stick.

Hints
1 Occasionally, it is useful to put the suction probe in the lateral port and aspirate the hepatorenal fossa or pararenal fossa.
2 Retract the laparoscope and camera a little while washing.
3 Where clot is present, irrigate with heparinized saline and mix the clot up with the saline using the probe. It can then be aspirated more easily. Attempts to aspirate unwashed clot result in a blocked sucker.

Clips
The types of clips available are described in Chapter 2, p. 24.

Technique
It is important to clean the structure to be occluded thoroughly first.

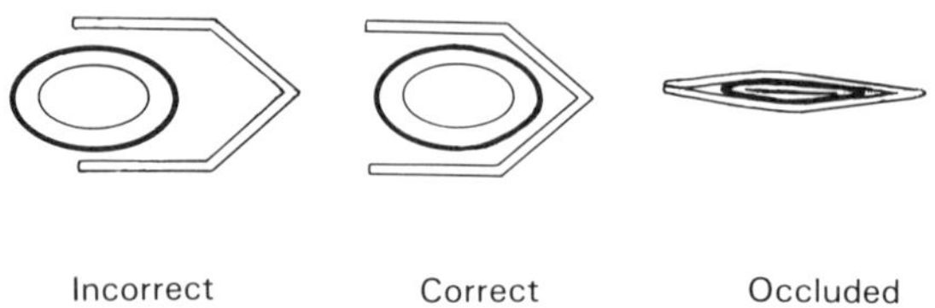

Fig. 4.14 Clips must be applied correctly or they will slip off.

Retract it away from neighbouring structures. Remove enough areolar tissue to make it possible to apply the size of clip available. Make sure you can see the distal end of the clip beyond the structure when applying (Fig. 4.14).

Multifire clip applicator
When this is used, a clip is loaded either automatically or by pressing the loading lever, according to design. Viewing the instrument through the laparoscope, note that the clip is loaded. Apply it, paying attention to the precautions as above, and close the jaws. A new clip can then be loaded without withdrawing the instrument.

Dangers
1 If there is tissue between the distal end of the clip, it is not properly applied and can be displaced or come off altogether (Fig. 4.14).
2 It can be very difficult to reapply a clip to a structure once its continuity has been divided.

Hints
1 The secret of safe clipping is to clean the structure thoroughly and observe that the clip is being applied correctly. It is also advisable to use a second clip on the patient side of structures such as the cystic duct and cystic artery.
2 Clips can be removed by grasping the angle of the clip and pulling in the line of application. They will then slide off (Fig. 4.15).

Self-locking clips (Fig. 4.16)
These are absorbable and unlike metallic clips will not hold their position once closed unless a locking device is engaged at the tips of the clip. They require a special clip applicator with a semi-closed and fully closed position. Insert the clip into the jaws, then semi-close the instrument. This allows it to pass down the cannula. Apply it to the

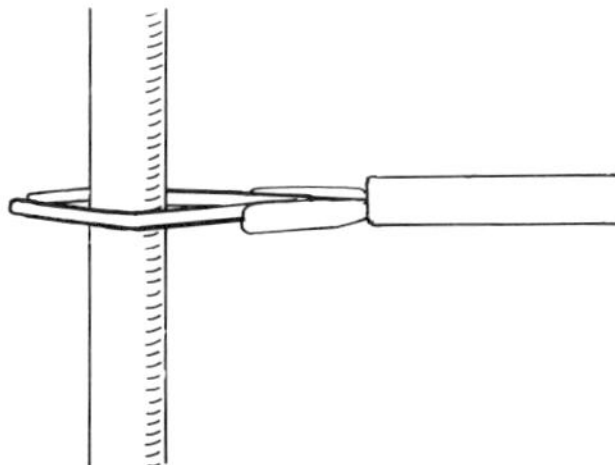

Fig. 4.15 Removing a metal clip.

vessel. Make sure the clipping mechanism is fully visible beyond the distal edge of the vessel. Close completely.

Dangers
If the vessel has not been adequately cleaned, tissue may get in the clipping mechanism and the clip will then come off.

Hints
Make sure the structure is fully dissected and clean before applying the clip. Do not try to apply a locking clip to a structure that is too large for it.

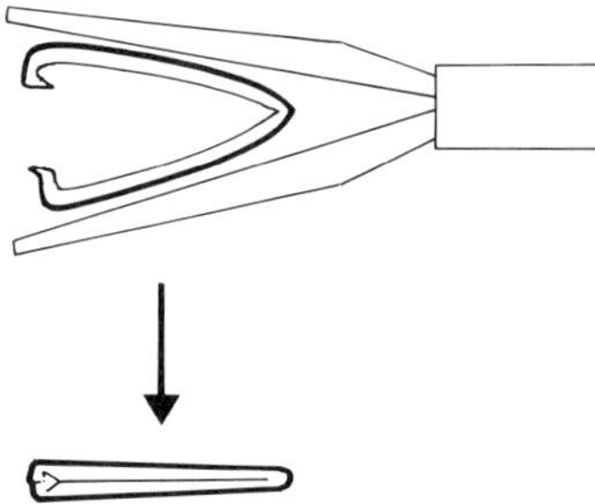

Fig. 4.16 Absorbable clips have a self-locking device at one end.

Tying knots and suturing

External knotting (Roeder knot)

Technique
In cases where it is not possible to safely occlude a vessel or duct with a clip, an alternative is to tie a ligature or use a preformed ligature. In 1918, Roeder described a sliding knot for use during tonsillectomy in children. This knot (Fig. 4.17) slides closed, but will not slide open.

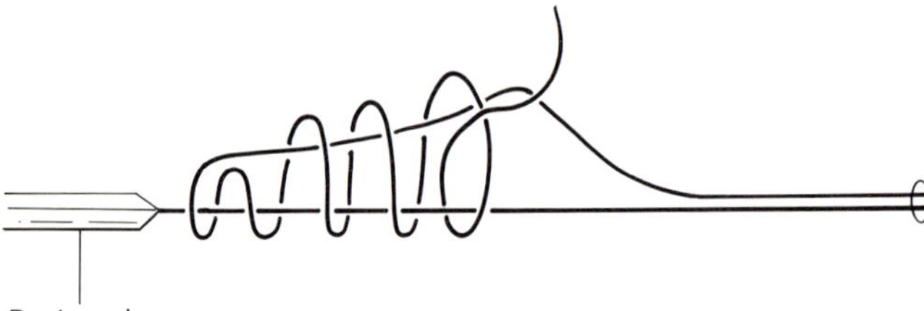

Fig. 4.17 The method of tying a Roeder knot.

It can either be tied at the time of surgery, or a preformed knot can be used. Catgut is the best suture material to use for this knot since it undergoes swelling once applied, thus further securing itself.

To tie a Roeder knot use a suitable instrument to take a catgut ligature down a port. Keep hold of the distal end. Loop the catgut around the structure to be ligated and retrieve the loose end. Bring it back out of the same cannula. Tie an external knot as in Fig. 4.17. Place a push tube on the catgut. Push the knot down into place and tighten it. Cut off the excess.

Dangers
Excessive traction may cause the structure to part. It can then be very difficult to retrieve the loose end.

Hints
1 When tying the knot outside a port, place the index finger of your left hand over the port and between the threads, so as to prevent the knot sliding down prematurely. It can then be tightened onto your finger.
2 When using the push rod, keep the ligature loop away from the structure itself until it is almost completely closed. Then position the loop and knot, if necessary using another grasper or dissecting forceps to position the tie, before finally tightening it.

Preformed catgut ligature
This is a pretied Roeder knot and is supplied prepacked and sterilized by the Ethicon Suture Company as an 'Ethibinder'. It is presented as a pretied loop mounted on a push rod. It can only be passed around a structure which has already been divided.

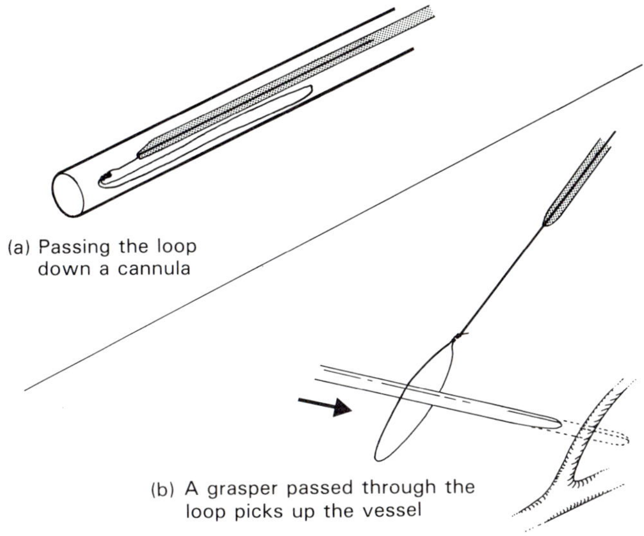

(a) Passing the loop
down a cannula

(b) A grasper passed through the
loop picks up the vessel

Fig. 4.18 The method of applying a preformed catgut loop ligature.

Technique

Divide the structure. Insert the loop via an introducer allowing the loop to trail behind the knot within the introducer. Push the preformed catgut ligature into the abdomen until the loop is free. Pass a grasper through the loop and pick up the structure to be ligated. Break the push rod at the preformed fracture site. Using the free pusher, push the knot down until it is almost closed. Position it exactly (Fig. 4.18). Complete closure of the loop. Insert scissors and cut off the excess end (Fig. 4.19).

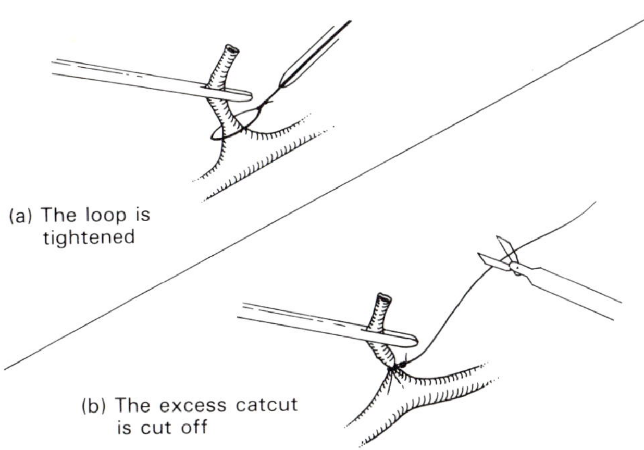

(a) The loop is
tightened

(b) The excess catcut
is cut off

Fig. 4.19 Tightening the knot.

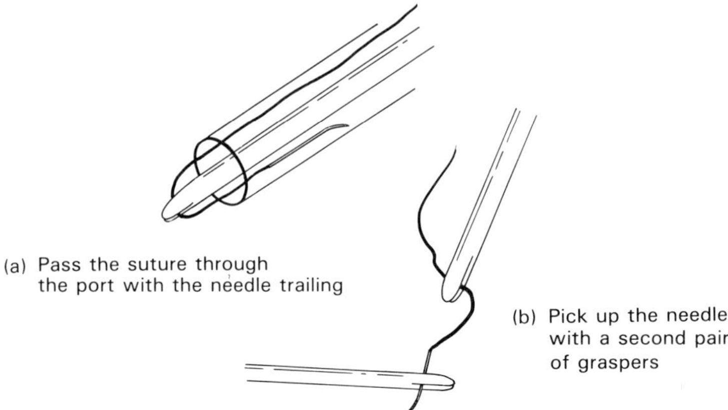

Fig. 4.20 Passing a suture into the abdomen.

Suturing

Needle holders and needles are described on pp. 20–1, 24.

Technique

Pick up the thread next to the needle. Pass it down a port allowing
the needle to trail behind the jaws of the grasping forceps (Fig. 4.20).
Pick up the needle with a second forceps from another port. Transfer
the needle back to the needle holder in a satisfactory orientation. Pass
the suture through the tissues and pull it almost through (Fig. 4.21).
Pick up the needle end of the thread and then tie a knot as described
above. Cut off the excess thread. Be careful not to drop the loose
needle.

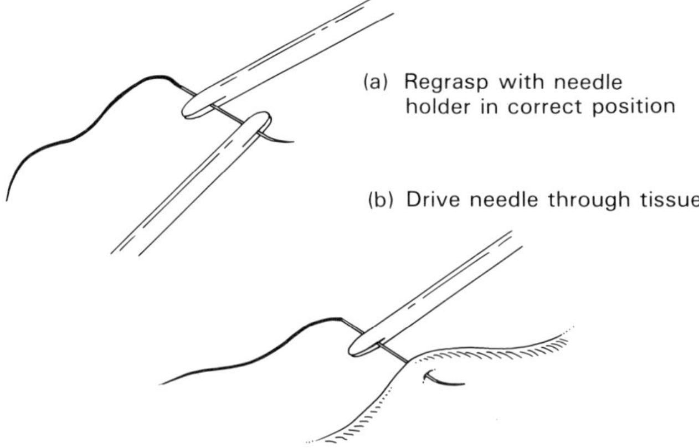

Fig. 4.21 The needle is grasped in the correct orientation and passed through
the tissue.

Dangers
It is easy to perforate vessels and other structures when the needle is being manipulated. It is essential to master this technique fully in a simulator before attempting it in a patient.

If the two throws of the knot are tied in the same direction, a slip knot will be produced which will later come undone.

The problem
There is difficulty in getting the angle of the needle right.

Hints
1 Use graspers to hold the tissues to be sutured and to move them at the correct angle to the needle.
2 If the suture site is on the abdominal wall, use external pressure to deform the wall and bring it into a suitable position for suturing.
3 In open surgery it is usual to move the needle to the tissues to be sutured. In laparoscopic surgery you have to be prepared to move the tissue to the site of the needle.

Notes
Loss of a needle in the peritoneum, see Chapter 9, p. 124.

Internal knots
These are particularly useful when a suture has been inserted laparoscopically and the ends are to be tied. The technique is illustrated in Figs 4.22 and 4.23.

Technique
Pick up one of the loose ends with a suitable forceps. Loop that end twice around another pair of forceps and pick up the other loose end with the same forceps. Draw one through the other creating a double half hitch. Tie the second throw of the knot using the opposite rotation of the forceps.

Dangers
The knot may slip open during the tying of the second throw.

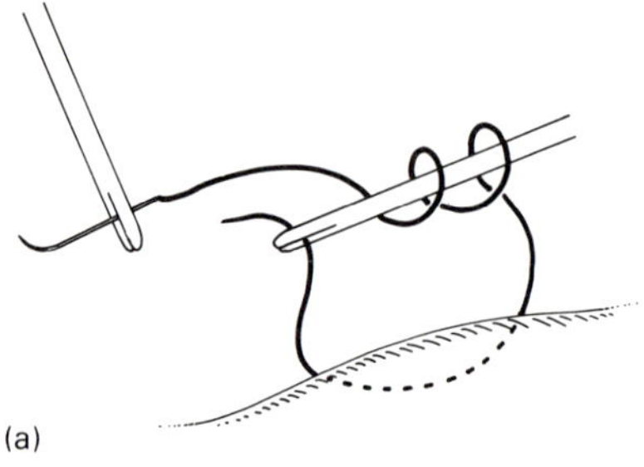

(a)

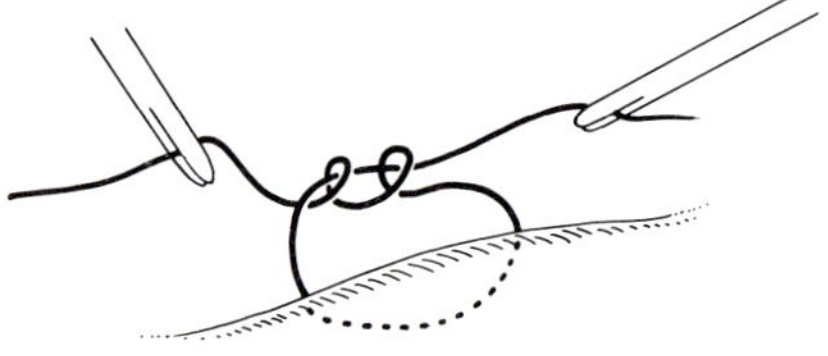

(b) First throw completed

Fig. 4.22 Stages of tying an internal knot.

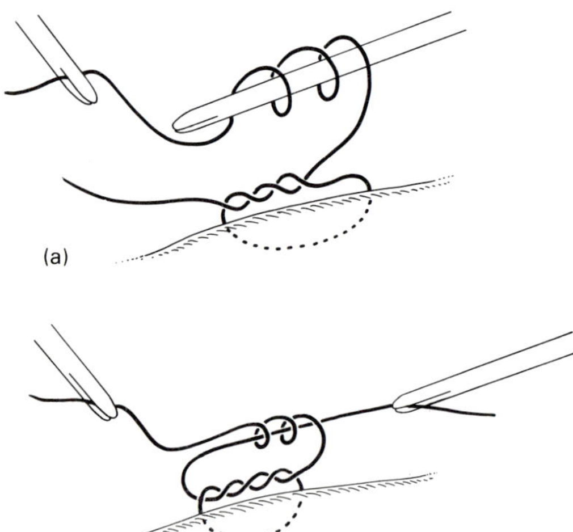

(a)

(b) Second throw completed

Fig. 4.23 The second throw is completed.

Hints

1 It is easier to tie knots with a forceps with curved tips. These prevent the half hitches from falling off as the next part of the knot is tied.

2 It can be useful to apply a metal clip to the ligature to maintain tension whilst the knot is being tied (Fig. 4.24).

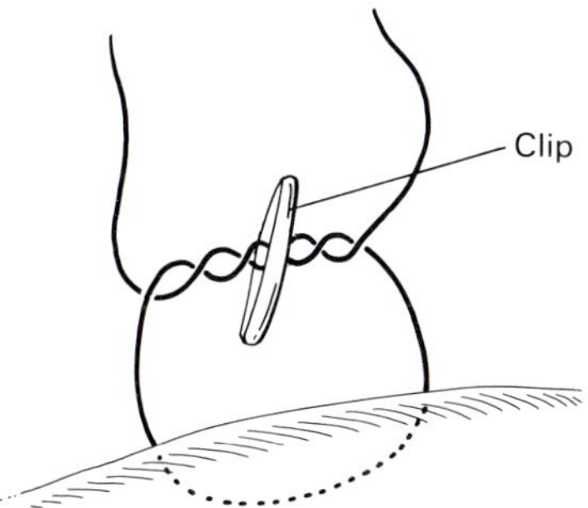

Fig. 4.24 Using a clip to prevent slippage of the first throw of a knot while the second is tied.

5: Pre-operative preparation

History and examination
Investigations
  Ultrasound
  Oral cholecystogram
  Liver function tests
  Endoscopic cholangiography
  Intravenous cholangiography
Patient preparation
  Laxative suppositories
  Shaving

Premedication
Bladder emptying
Deep vein thrombosis prophylaxis
Antibiotic prophylaxis
Informed consent
  Possibility of open cholecystectomy
  Choledocholithiasis
  Video tapes
  Recovery

History and examination

In addition to assessing the patient's general condition and anaesthetic risk factors, try to establish whether the symptoms are likely to be due to gallstones or not. Occasionally atypical symptoms can persist after the removal of a gallbladder containing stones and it is valuable to point out this possibility to the patient before the operation is undertaken. Persistent symptoms are otherwise likely to be blamed on the operation itself.

Make an assessment of the severity of the disease in the gallbladder. This may help to indicate how much operative time will be required. In particular, establish whether the patient has recently been jaundiced or had pancreatitis, as this will indicate the need for a pre-operative endoscopic cholangiogram and possibly a sphincterotomy.

Factors in the history and examination which may indicate a more difficult operation include the following.

1 A long history of multiple severe attacks.

2 A very recent severe attack of acute cholecystitis. It has been our practice to wait 6 weeks after the last symptoms subside as laparoscopic cholecystectomy is likely to be more difficult if the gallbladder is still inflamed.

3 Jaundice or pancreatitis. Persistent jaundice, a recent history of jaundice, or pancreatitis suggest possible stones in the common bile duct.

4 Previous peritonitis.

5 Previous abdominal surgery, particularly in the upper abdomen. Previous upper abdominal surgery is a relative contraindication to the novice, since the resultant adhesions complicate laparoscopic surgery. Lower abdominal surgery is less likely to leave complex adhesions.

6 Abdominal scars. Ascertain any history of postoperative sepsis,

wound dehiscence or reoperation as these may indicate more severe adhesions.

7 Significant tenderness over the gallbladder.

8 Spinal kyphosis. This can make access difficult, particularly in thin elderly patients.

Investigations

Ultrasound

We use ultrasonography routinely to diagnose gallbladder disease. It is not good at identifying common bile duct stones. Indicators of possible operative difficulty include the following.

1 Thickening of the gallbladder wall persisting between acute attacks of inflammation (more than 3 mm).

2 A stone stuck in Hartmann's pouch close to the bile duct.

3 Large gallstones (greater than 1.5 cm in diameter).

4 Dilated common bile duct (more than 10 mm). This may indicate stones in the common duct and an endoscopic cholangiogram is indicated.

5 An intrahepatic gallbladder.

6 Gallbladder packed with stones.

Easier gallbladders may be indicated by the following.

1 A thin-walled gallbladder distended with fluid.

2 A few small stones.

3 Gallbladder on a subhepatic mesentery.

None of these indicators are absolutely reliable but they can be helpful in planning an operating list. It is useful to educate the ultrasonographer to look for these signs.

Oral cholecystogram

We rarely use this investigation now. If one is available, it may give a clear indication of whether the gallbladder is still functioning. A non-functioning gallbladder with a thick wall is likely to be more difficult to remove. It also gives a clear picture of the site, size, and mobility of the stones, and may show the length and insertion of the cystic duct.

Liver function tests

Recent or persistently abnormal liver function tests especially raised bilirubin and alkaline phosphatase may indicate a persistent stone in the biliary tree, and the need for pre-operative endoscopic cholangiography.

Endoscopic cholangiography (ERCP)

The side viewing endoscope used for endoscopic cholangiography can also be used therapeutically to clear stones from a duct by sphincterotomy and balloon or Dormia basket extraction. It is our practice to refer patients for endoscopic cholangiography and sphincterotomy where there is a suspicion of common duct stones.

Some surgeons advocate this investigation as a way of avoiding a peroperative cholangiogram. An ERCP gives a 'road map' of the biliary tree and can give useful information about the length and insertion of the cystic duct. An operative cholangiogram, on the other hand, shows the site of cannulation and tells the surgeon where he or she is 'on the map' before irretrievable damage is done. Also, stones occasionally enter the bile duct during the delay between an ERCP and cholecystectomy, or even during the operation itself.

We carry out an operative cholangiogram whether an ERCP is available or not.

Intravenous cholangiography

We favour ERCP rather than intravenous cholangiography which is less accurate, not therapeutic and carries its own risks (e.g. 1 in 4000 rate of life-threatening anaphylaxis).

Patient preparation

Laxative suppositories

The patient should be given two 5 mg bisacodyl suppositories (Dulcolax, Boehringer Ingelheim Ltd) to use the evening prior to surgery. These encourage evacuation of colonic contents, thus improving the laparoscopic view over the transverse colon from the umbilicus to Calot's triangle.

Shaving

After clerking on the ward the patient is shaved as for a laparotomy, from nipples to pubis. Not all surgeons advocate this but we prefer to keep hairs away from the abdominal wounds.

Premedication

The premedication is the province of the anaesthetist (see Chapter 6), but we feel strongly that an analgesic suppository such as 100 mg diclofenac (Voltarol, Geigy Pharmaceuticals) given 1 hour prior to surgery improves postoperative recovery.

Bladder emptying

Prior to insertion of the Verres needle the bladder should be emptied to avoid inadvertent damage. This can be satisfactorily achieved in most patients by asking them to void immediately prior to surgery. However, men over 60 years should be formally catheterized (under full aseptic precautions), because of the possibility of bladder outflow obstruction and consequently urinary retention. Indeed all patients may be catheterized at the start of the operation as a precaution, and the catheter removed once the bladder is empty. There is no need to leave an indwelling catheter for the duration of surgery, since the bladder is only at risk during insertion of the Verres needle and the peri-umbilical cannula.

Deep vein thrombosis prophylaxis

We do not routinely give heparin prophylaxis to patients undergoing laparoscopic cholecystectomy though the patients do receive a small dose of heparin through the irrigation fluid used intraperitoneally. Patients are fitted with antithrombosis stockings for the duration of the operation, and encouraged to be up and mobile after surgery. Because patients are not tied to intravenous drips or in pain, they mobilize quickly and fully, and thrombo-embolic complications are unusual. Moreover, haemorrhage is a major problem in laparoscopic surgery and avoidance of anticoagulation is desirable.

Antibiotic prophylaxis

We give a single dose of a third generation cephalosporin (2 g cefotaxime) intravenously at the start of surgery. This ensures maximum plasma levels peri-operatively. Alternatively, the antibiotic could be given intramuscularly with the premedication. We do not routinely continue the antibiotics beyond the first dose. (The only exception to this rule was a patient immunosuppressed for a heart transplant who had an empyema of the gallbladder removed laparoscopically.)

Informed consent

Prior to surgery all our patients are given an advice sheet to read which describes the operation and its potential complications (see Appendix).

Possibility of open cholecystectomy

It is important to stress that while every effort will be made to perform the operation laparoscopically this cannot be guaranteed, and the decision to convert to an open operation must be left to the surgeon at the time of surgery.

Choledocholithiasis

The patient is informed that an operative cholangiogram will be performed if possible. If it indicates that stones are present then an attempt to remove them will be made or they will be left for a subsequent ERCP, whichever is the local practice. If stone removal would be deferred to ERCP the patient should be counselled that open exploration of the common bile duct may still be required if ERCP fails.

Video tapes

Video tapes of the operation are excellent teaching aids for the surgeon, and provide an invaluable record if postoperative problems do occur. We do not give patients copies of their video tapes since these contain long periods of irrelevant material, and require a lot of time for explanation if they are to be of value to the patient. Otherwise they are subject to misinterpretation. We simply do not have the resources both to treat the patient and indulge in this time-consuming activity.

Recovery

Finally, the patient should be told about the expected rapid recovery, so that both patient and relatives can be ready for discharge later the same day or the following day.

Relatives should also be reassured that early activity is not dangerous and should be encouraged. Unless they are told this directly, our experience suggests that some will delay the patient's recovery by being overprotective.

6: Anaesthesia for laparoscopic cholecystectomy*

Pre-operative management
  General
  Premedication
Operative management
  Bradycardia
  Heat loss
  Muscle relaxation
  Raised intra-abdominal pressure
  Potential for gas embolus
  Potential for haemorrhage
  Gastric distension
Bladder
Position and patient safety
Other drugs
Postoperative management
  Wound pain
  Shoulder pain
  Nausea
  Shivering
Summary of key features of
    anaesthetic management

Pre-operative management

General

The more significant the medical problems of the patient, the greater the advantage of using the laparoscopic rather than the open technique of cholecystectomy. In particular, the postoperative period is curtailed and less stressed because of minimal pain and early mobilization. This means that many patients can have significant medical disease and assessment that fitness is optimal must be made carefully.

The principles of management are the same for open as for laparoscopic — for instance, the grossly obese should lose weight. Where this is not possible, they will be suitable for either technique, though different surgical problems are posed. Postoperatively, there is clear advantage to the laparoscopic group as regards all forms of pre-existing medical problems.

Premedication

Pre-operative sedation will be appreciated by a patient who has had little time to settle into the ward before surgery.

A short-acting benzodiazepine (e.g. temazepam) and a long-acting non-steroidal anti-inflammatory drug (NSAID, e.g. diclofenac) orally have proved useful.

Hints

1 If patients are brought into hospital only briefly before surgery, assessment must be done in a pre-anaesthetic clinic.

2 Although restlessness in the early postoperative period can be reduced by the use of heavier pre-operative sedation with longer

*This chapter has been contributed by Dr M.J. Lindop.

acting agents, patients response is unpredictable and it is preferable to use shorter acting agents in modest dosage to achieve a consistently rapid recovery.

Operative management

General anaesthesia is required with tracheal intubation and positive pressure ventilation. Techniques suitable for routine laparotomies are appropriate but there are several specific factors that need to be addressed. Key factors are a light plane of anaesthesia to allow rapid recovery following abrupt completion of surgery, and careful monitoring of ventilation by use of both pulse oximetry and end-tidal carbon dioxide measurement.

Bradycardia

The time between induction of anaesthesia and induction of the pneumoperitoneum may be half an hour because of draping and the connection of equipment. The depressant effect of induction drugs will be fully revealed with no compensatory surgical stimulus. A slow heart rate is often seen. When peritoneal insufflation begins, vagal stimulation further drops the rate.

Hints
The occurrence of bradycardia is so common that the prophylactic use of atropine should be considered.

Heat loss

Although intra-operative loss may be less than for an open cholecystectomy because the peritoneum is not exposed, the prolonged induction/setting-up phase can allow considerable unnecessary loss due to careless exposure before surgery has even started. Cooling delays and impairs recovery.

Hints
1 Overblankets should not be removed until the 'last minute'. The problems with water blankets and operative cholangiography have been much overstated, and blankets are now available without linear flow pipes. We use a warming blanket routinely. Falls in temperature intra-operatively may be reduced to less than $1°C$ by careful management.
2 Temperature monitoring increases awareness of the problem.

Muscle relaxation

Muscle relaxation is essential and improves the compliance of the abdominal cavity. Insufflation is normally controlled automatically to maintain a constant intra-abdominal pressure (10–14 mmHg) so that the volume of gas contained (and therefore the working space apparent to the surgeon) is increased by good relaxation. In patients without strong musculature, use of muscle relaxants may be minimal if apnoea can be maintained by an adequate plane of anaesthesia and associated respiratory inhibition.

Hints

1 It is helpful to monitor neuromuscular blockade, for where recovery of neuromuscular function has occurred, the use of neostigmine (a contributor to postoperative nausea) may not be necessary.
2 The choice of a short-acting non-depolarizing muscle relaxant (e.g. atracurium, vecuronium), reduces the problems posed by the operative difficulties which can vary greatly. The procedure can move very quickly from a difficult and slow dissection of a gallbladder bed through rapid extraction of the freed gallbladder to completion of surgery, or each of these latter stages may be prolonged.

Raised intra-abdominal pressure

Maintenance of the pneumoperitoneum is essential to allow the surgeon space to operate. The automatic insufflation of carbon dioxide to a predetermined pressure is usually trouble free. However, the anaesthetist must be on guard against equipment failure leading to overinflation. Rise in airway pressure or reduction in ventilation volume can ensue. Reduction of functional residual capacity will impair gas exchange and may lead to hypoxaemia. Venous return will be impaired and blood pressure and cardiac output falls further aggravate the hypoxic state.

Hints

Where a vent circuit is used to recycle gas and clean the smoke, inaccuracies will occur when the pressure is monitored on a side arm of this circuit. A separate pressure monitor/insufflator line is strongly recommended. The circulator must not be used unless the pressure line is connected and functioning. (Further discussion is in Chapter 1, p. 11.)

Potential for gas embolus

Gas may be accidentally infused directly by vessel puncture with the Verres needle. It may also arise from the pneumoperitoneum. Contributing factors will be low venous pressure and failure of cut veins to collapse in the usual manner when they are held open by surrounding tissue fibrosis.

Hints

1 Fluids should be given to prevent hypovolaemia.
2 Continuous monitoring of end-tidal carbon dioxide is essential as a sudden fall gives early warning of significant gas embolism.
3 Where the gas embolus is soluble carbon dioxide the effect should be short-lived; if air has been entrained into the pneumoperitoneum from a leak in the vent circuit, the problem may be more prolonged.
4 Remedial action will include:
   (a) identifying the cause,
   (b) increasing venous pressure,
   (c) tilting the patient head down,
   (d) switching off the insufflation,
   (e) desufflating the abdomen, and
   (f) withdrawing nitrous oxide.

Potential for haemorrhage

Although blood loss is usually trivial, good (16 gauge) venous access is essential to allow rapid replacement of lost fluid. Assessment of loss is difficult because significant amounts of blood may remain in the peritoneal cavity at the end of the procedure in the pelvis or the paracolic gutters, and because the blood sucked out will be diluted by saline wash. Sites of potential loss include mesenteric vessels (damaged at laparoscopy), unusually large vessels in the gallbladder bed, and the major vessels of the porta hepatis. Where anatomy is normal and scarring minimal, problems are rare. Other major vessels may be damaged especially where specialized insufflation techniques are used when scars and adhesions prohibit the routine approach.

Hints

If major bleeding is seen, early laparotomy is advisable. Blood is normally grouped and saved for these patients.

Gastric distension

Gastric distension will obscure the view of the gallbladder. It may be present pre-operatively or may have been induced by problems with ventilating the lungs prior to tracheal intubation.

Hints

A large (18 gauge) oro-gastric tube should be passed. This can be done after induction and prior to tracheal intubation.

Bladder

Prior to laparoscopy it is safer to drain the bladder. Although operations now rarely last more than 2 hours, it is convenient to place an indwelling catheter. Alternatively, the patient may be asked to void urine immediately before the operation, or the bladder may be emptied by transient catheterization at the start of surgery.

Hints

1 The drainage bag should be led to the head of the table to allow monitoring of urine production.
2 An indwelling catheter is removed at the end of surgery.

Position and patient safety

Visualization of the gallbladder is helped by using head-up tilt with left lateral roll. Too extreme a position must be avoided, with care taken to prevent pressure area damage. Hypotension may occur. The eyes are securely taped and covered to prevent accidental damage when laser probes are in use.

Other drugs

Prophylactic antibiotics, e.g. cefotaxime, are routinely and conveniently given intravenously after induction of anaesthesia.

Postoperative management

The lungs are maximally inflated prior to deflating the abdomen. The anaesthetic is discontinued and the muscle relaxant antagonized. An anti-emetic (e.g. metoclopramide) is injected intravenously. Analgesia is established. The four wound sites are infiltrated locally each with about 5 ml 0.25% bupivicaine. Alternatively, or additionally, the right-sided intercostal nerves are blocked from T6 to T11 in the midaxillary line with 18 ml 0.25% bupivicaine. Systemic analgesics may be required depending on the effectiveness of the local anaesthesia. There is also pain arising from the peritoneum, most noticeable if a drain is left in the gallbladder bed. Incremental doses of pethidine, or equivalent, can help to settle patients when first awakening.

Wound pain

Any pain rapidly subsides and it is all too easy to prescribe unnecessarily high doses of narcotic analgesics. Patient controlled analgesia has not proved helpful. Excessive narcotic analgesics contribute to nausea which remains the dominant postoperative problem.

Hints

1 The use of NSAIDs can reduce narcotic analgesic requirements.
2 Patients can take oral analgesics unless they are nauseated.

Shoulder pain

Diaphragmatic irritation is another source of pain, usually arising later in the postoperative period.

Hints

Maximum inflation of the lungs as gas is evacuated from the abdomen at the end of surgery will reduce the remaining volume, and lessen the risk of this pain.

Nausea

Nausea is a dominant postoperative problem. The combination of side effects of anaesthetic and analgesic drugs with prolonged peritoneal traction gives a significant incidence.

Hints

1 Anaesthetic technique should be planned with avoidance of nausea as a high priority. Anti-emetics, e.g. metoclopramide, are given intravenously at the end of surgery.
2 Small doses of droperidol and other anti-emetic strategies should be explored.
3 Limiting the use of narcotic analgesics will help.
4 Pre-operative discussion of the problem with the patient can

change their perception of pain and reduce their need for narcotic analgesics with their attendant risk of nausea.

Shivering

Shivering increases the risk of postoperative hypoxia (a nauseant factor) and slows recovery. Measures to avoid heat loss should be applied carefully, and recovery rooms should be warm.

Summary of key features of anaesthetic management

1 Optimal pre-operative fitness.
2 Light premedication.
3 Good venous access.
4 End-tidal carbon dioxide monitoring (ventilation, embolus).
5 Beware of bradycardia.
6 Oro-gastric tube to manage gastric dilatation.
7 Check intra-abdominal pressure monitoring.
8 Short-acting muscle relaxants.
9 Maximally inflate the lungs when pneumoperitoneum emptied.
10 Establish good postoperative analgesia.
11 Prevent nausea.

7: The operation of laparoscopic cholecystectomy

Anatomy
  Normal anatomy
  Important variations in anatomy
Setting up
  Position of patient
  Layout of theatre
  Setting up theatre
  Preparation of the skin
  Sterile connections
  Testing routines
The operation
  Inserting the operative ports
    First port
    Second port
    Third port
    Fourth port
  Exposure of Calot's triangle

Retraction of the gallbladder
Adhesions to the gallbladder
Defining the cystic duct
Cholangiogram
The cystic artery
Freeing the gallbladder from
  its bed
The gallbladder bed
Inserting a drain
Haemostasis
Peritoneal toilet
Extracting the gallbladder
Use of a bag for extraction
Enlarging the exit port
Closing the linea alba
Closing the skin

Anatomy

Normal anatomy (Fig. 7.1)

In order to undertake laparoscopic cholecystectomy it is mandatory to be thoroughly familiar with the relevant anatomy and possible variations. This is even more important than for open cholecystectomy as the anatomy is encountered from an unfamiliar aspect during laparoscopy.

The gallbladder lies under the right lobe of the liver to which it may be attached directly or by a mesentery. Alternatively, it may be almost completely embedded within the liver substance (intrahepatic gallbladder). The fundus of the gallbladder may extend out to the liver edge or be confined within the lower border of the right lobe of the liver. Medially, the gallbladder usually narrows slightly to form Hartmann's pouch from which the cystic duct drains. In general, the duct arises from the upper left side of the pouch, rather than the apparent apex of the gallbladder, though it may come off at a variety of positions and angles. There may be a gradual tapering of Hartmann's pouch straight into the cystic duct or more often the pouch may be very wide and suddenly narrow into a small cystic duct. A bulky Hartmann's pouch may overlie the cystic duct itself. The cystic duct then joins the common hepatic duct to form the common bile duct, classically opening into the right edge of that structure, just above the duodenum.

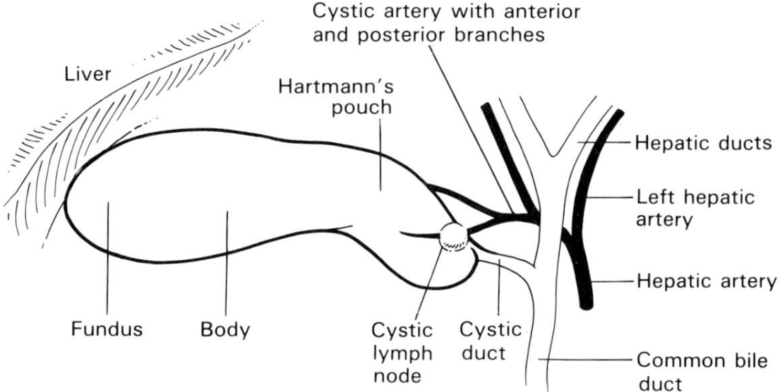

Fig. 7.1 Schematic diagram of 'normal' gallbladder anatomy.

The hepatic artery usually lies posterior to the common bile duct (76% of cases) and after bifurcating the right hepatic branch runs parallel with the cystic duct and medial edge of the gallbladder. The cystic artery classically comes off the right hepatic artery (95% of cases), to the right of the common hepatic duct, and divides into an anterior and posterior branch to supply the gallbladder wall. The cystic lymph node lies over the anterior cystic artery, where it crosses the cystic duct (Fig. 7.1).

Summary of technique with standard anatomy

First define and clip the cystic duct. After performing a cholangiogram and dividing the cystic duct, clip and divide the main stem of the cystic artery. Lift the gallbladder away from the gallbladder bed and remove it.

Important variations in anatomy

Although there are many known anatomical variations some are particularly misleading in laparoscopic cholecystectomy and will be mentioned here.

Bile ducts

THE CYSTIC DUCT IS VERY SHORT

This is particularly dangerous if it is obscured by an overlying Hartmann's pouch. If there are adhesions and fibrosis, a small common bile duct may then look like the cystic duct (Fig. 7.2).

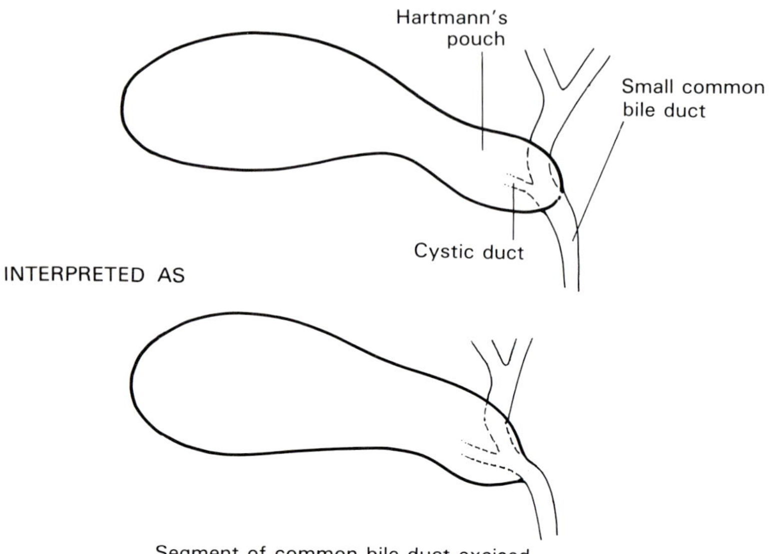

Fig. 7.2 With a short cystic duct behind Hartmann's pouch, opening into a small common bile duct, the common bile duct may be mistaken for the cystic duct.

Dangers
The common bile duct is mistakenly opened or divided.

Hints
1 Be quite certain you have seen that the gallbladder narrows down into the cystic duct before clipping or dividing medially.
2 Make certain there is no cranially running duct arising from the upper edge or posterior aspect of the supposed 'cystic duct'.

THE CYSTIC DUCT IS VERY SHORT AND ENTERS THE RIGHT HEPATIC DUCT
The continuation of the right hepatic duct is often posterior and out of view (Fig. 7.3). The origin of the right hepatic duct can be mistaken for the cystic duct.

Dangers
The right hepatic duct is divided.

Hints
1 Always encircle the cystic duct close to Hartmann's pouch. If it is

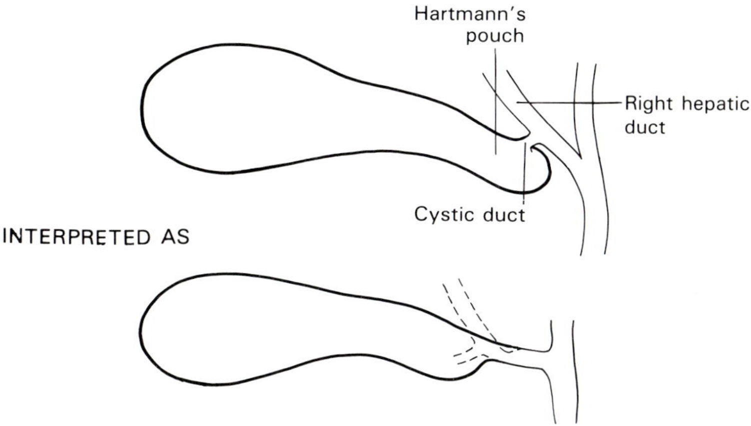

Fig. 7.3 With a short cystic duct opening into the right hepatic duct, the right hepatic duct may be mistaken for the cystic duct.

difficult to go round the duct it may be because there is a continuation of the right hepatic duct coming off posteriorly.

2 If in doubt, move further up the gallbladder itself keeping very close to its wall. Go round it and then extend the dissection medially, retracting the gallbladder away from the liver until the true cystic duct is seen.

THE CYSTIC DUCT IS LONG AND CROSSES THE COMMON DUCT ENTERING LOW DOWN ON ITS LATERAL ASPECT

See Figs 7.4 and 7.5.

Dangers

This is not usually a problem unless the isolation of the cystic duct

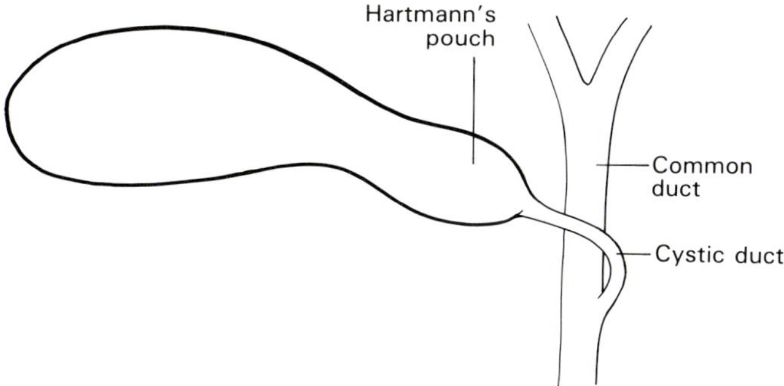

Fig. 7.4 A long cystic duct running across the common duct.

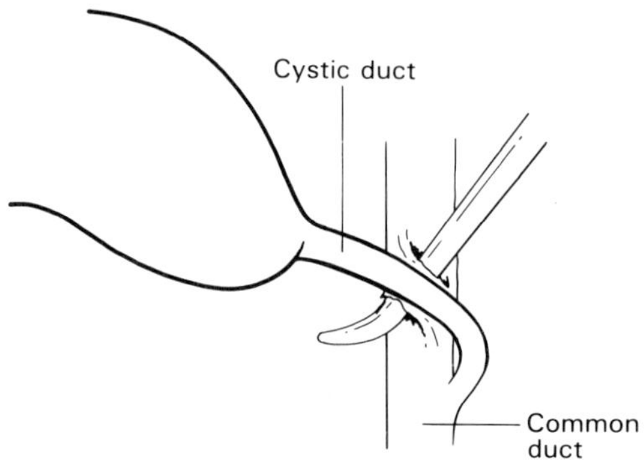

Fig. 7.5 If the cystic duct is adherent there is a danger of damage to the common duct behind it.

is carried out too far medially in which case there is a danger of damaging the common duct which lies posteriorly.

Hints
Always isolate the cystic duct close to the neck of the gallbladder. Do not worry about freeing the full length of the cystic duct but make sure there are no stones in it before inserting a cholangiogram catheter or dividing it. This can be done by gently squeezing the duct with atraumatic forceps from medial to lateral, milking any debris towards the opening in the cystic duct.

Arteries

ANTERIOR CYSTIC ARTERY (Fig. 7.6)
24% of cystic arteries run in front of the hepatic ducts, arising from a variety of sites.

This may be mistaken for the cystic duct (Fig. 7.7), but the error is usually apparent once it is divided. There may be another cystic artery lying posteriorly which is encountered later in the dissection.

Hints
Divide an anterior cystic artery first if it is obscuring the view.

SEVERAL SHORT CYSTIC ARTERIES ARISE FROM THE
RIGHT HEPATIC ARTERY

Dangers
The right hepatic artery may be divided in error believing it to be the

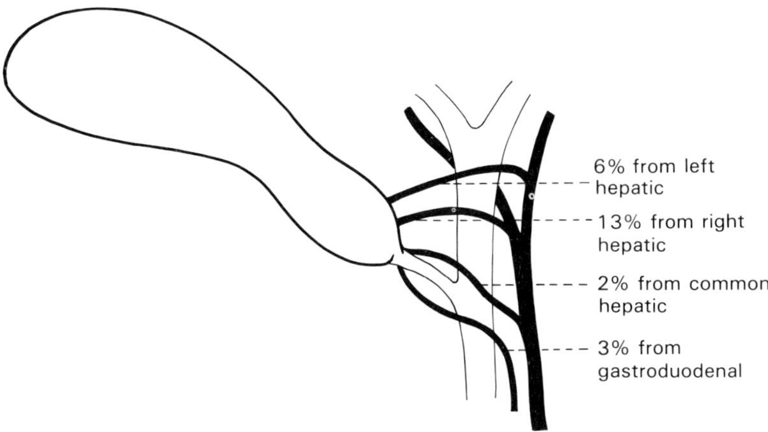

Fig. 7.6 24% of cystic arteries run in front of the hepatic ducts.

cystic artery. Even if this is not done dissection between the gall-bladder wall and the hepatic bed may result in haemorrhage from one of the more distal short cystic arteries.

Hints
Suspect that there is another cystic artery branch if the neck of the gallbladder will not pull away from the liver but still seems to be tethered. Dissect carefully. Isolate any further branches and clip them until the gallbladder becomes more mobile.

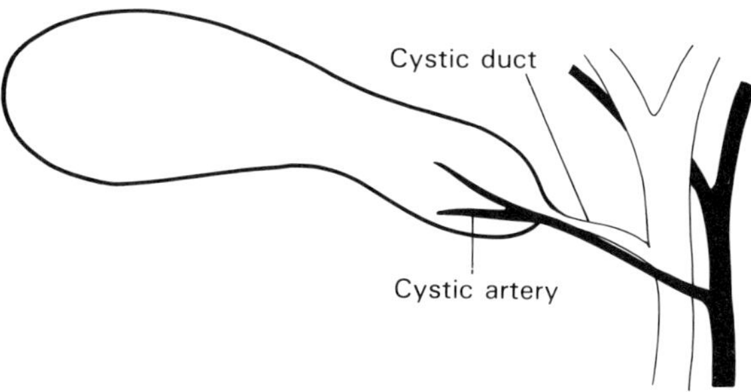

Fig. 7.7 An anterior cystic artery can be mistaken for the cystic duct.

SEPARATE ANTERIOR AND POSTERIOR CYSTIC ARTERIES COME OFF THE HEPATIC ARTERIES

The anomalous accessory cystic artery lies anteriorly, and is mistaken for the cystic artery trunk.

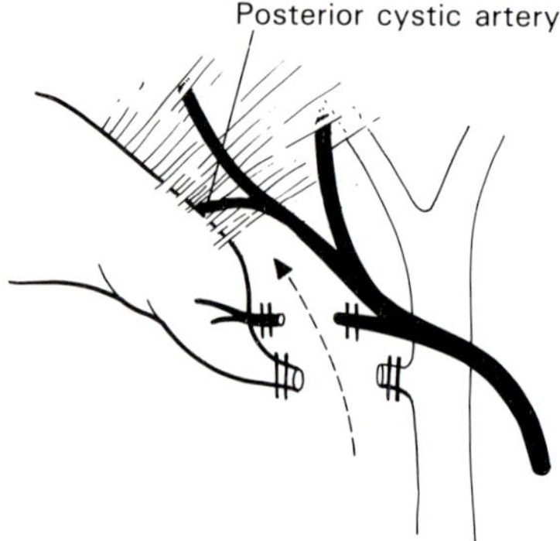

Fig. 7.8 A separate posterior cystic artery may be encountered as the gallbladder is excised from its bed. The main cystic artery may also occupy this position.

Dangers
The second posterior cystic artery is encountered as the gallbladder is being removed (Fig. 7.8) and results in major haemorrhage which obscures the view and may be difficult to control.

Hints
Always be suspicious of this anomaly and dissect the gallbladder from its bed carefully until it is clear there are no arteries remaining.

Setting up

Position of patient
The patient is placed supine on the operating table. It must be possible to tilt the table foot down and rotate it left side down. An X-ray cassette holder should be in position beneath the patient.

The anaesthetist is positioned at the patient's head with the anaesthetic machine on his or her right side. Monitors are placed at 45° angles in line with each of the patient's shoulders. The patient's arms are positioned by his or her side. Compressive stockings may be applied to the legs to increase venous return.

The surgeon stands on the patient's left facing the video screen beyond the patient's right shoulder. The assistant stands opposite the surgeon facing the other video screen. If only one video screen is available it should be moved closer to the head of the table with the anaesthetist's trolly on his or her left (Fig. 7.9).

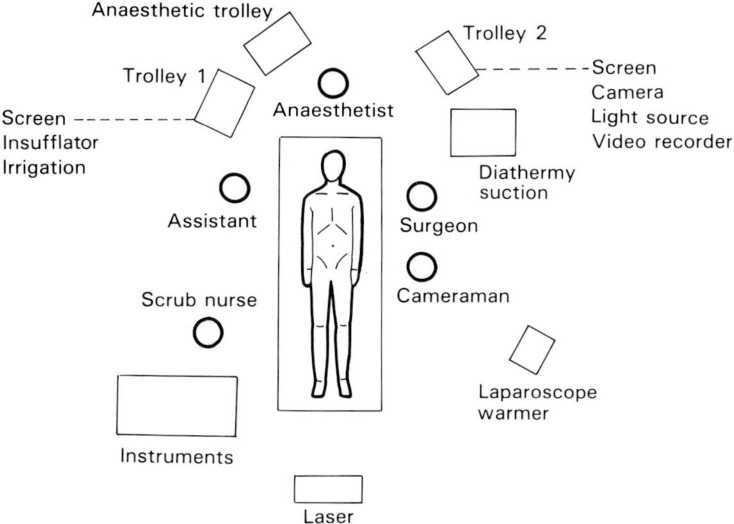

Fig. 7.9 The layout used in our operating theatre.

A variation in this position is known locally as the 'French position' (Fig. 7.10). The surgeon operates standing between the patient's legs and the patient is in a modified Lloyd Davies position as for an anterior resection of the rectum. Various other layouts are possible.

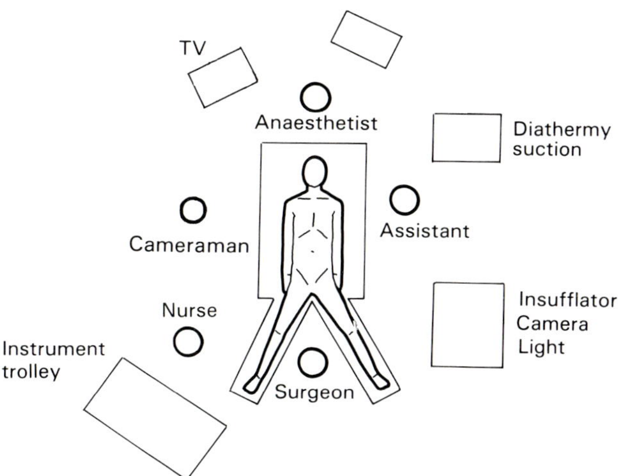

Fig. 7.10 An alternative layout with the surgeon seated between the patient's legs.

Layout of theatre

The insufflator is situated on the same trolley as the video screen on the patient's right. The suction and irrigation apparatus may also be on this trolley.

The video camera unit and light source are situated on the trolley underneath the video screen on the patient's left. The diathermy machine is also situated on this side.

The scrub nurse stands opposite the surgeon near the foot of the table with the instrument trolley on the patient's right at the level of the feet. The laser if used is situated at the end of the table near the patient's feet. The warming apparatus for the laparoscope is placed behind the surgeon and to his or her right.

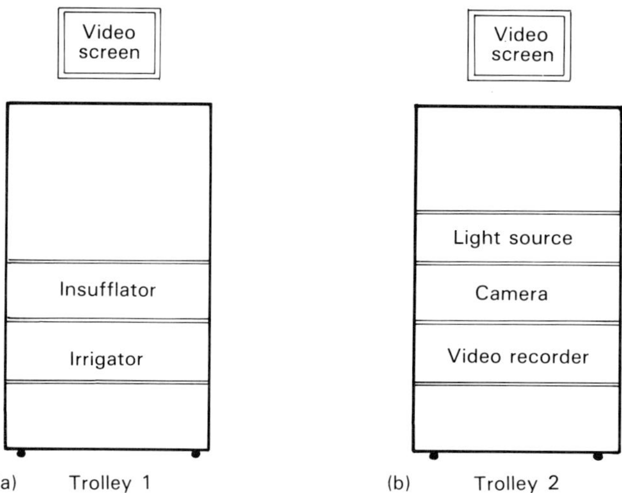

Fig. 7.11 Possible trolley arrangements.

Setting up theatre

At present a large number of items of theatre equipment need to be arranged, interconnected and attached to the operating table. It is probable that this number of interconnections will be simplified as technology improves.

The laparoscopy and video apparatus is best kept on pre-arranged trolleys. Our preferred arrangement is shown in Fig. 7.11 and 7.12 but many other variations are possible.

1 Move these trolleys into theatre with the connecting wires attached to the various units ready for joining up.

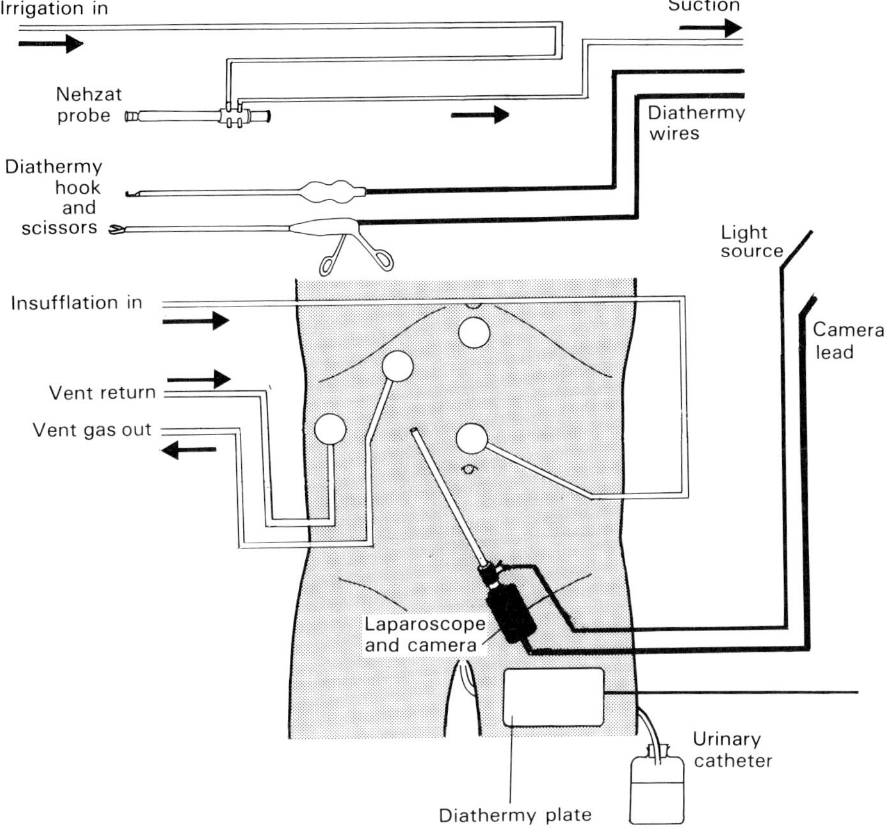

Fig. 7.12 Our preferred arrangement for the various tubes and wires connected to the patient and operating table.

2 Place the laparoscope in the sterile warming bath.

3 Anaesthesia is then induced and the patient positioned on the table.

4 If the patient has not voided prior to surgery a catheter should be inserted and the bladder emptied.

5 Connect the diathermy plate in the preferred position (e.g. on the patient's thigh) using the usual precautions to ensure there is good contact.

6 The equipment trolleys are moved into position and the interconnections made. The electrical circuits are connected supplying power to all items of equipment.

7 Video apparatus. The camera and monitors are connected to the video unit.

8 Suction irrigation. The system is connected up, pressurized and tested.

9 Insufflator. A fresh, full cylinder of carbon dioxide is attached.

10 Test insufflator. Check that there is adequate output flow and check the circuit for leaks (see pp. 79–80).

Preparation of the skin

Where required the skin will have been shaved pre-operatively. The skin is cleaned from nipples to groins with whatever antiseptic preparation is preferred. We use Betadine.

Apply sterile towels. The upper margin should be 2 cm above the xiphisternum, the lower margin should be at the level of the pubic symphysis. The left lateral towel should be lateral to the mid-clavicular line, the right lateral towel should be on a line just lateral to the anterior axillary line and iliac crest. We usually stick these towels on with adhesive tapes. This prevents wires and tubes falling between the towels and the patient, and does not interfere with the cholangiogram. It is not advisable to cover the whole abdomen with transparent film as pieces of the plastic may be carried into the peritoneal cavity on the tips of the trocars.

Sterile connections

Make the various sterile connections. Ensure the sterile end of wires, light source, and tubes are not 'handed out' and accidentally desterilized. It is useful to have a repeatable routine for this so that tubes and wires do not become entangled and nothing is forgotten. Our routine is as follows.

1 Gas in. The tubing bringing gas from the insufflator is brought across the patient's chest, down the left side of the abdomen and coiled over the patient's thighs.

2 Gas out (to recirculating pump). The gas exhaust tubing is brought in across the patient's right shoulder, passed down the right side of the abdomen and coiled over the patient's thighs. It is useful to mark these two tubes with different colours (e.g. yellow: gas in, red: exhaust gas) and mark their terminals on the machine similarly.

3 Vent return (from recirculating smoke extraction pump). The vent return tube is laid on the right side of the abdomen adjacent to the 'gas out' line.

4 Irrigation in. The line bringing pressurized heparinized saline from

the suction/irrigation apparatus is passed from the right side across the patient's chest and fixed through a clip on the left side of the chest. A suitable length of tubing is then attached to the suction/irrigation probe which is held in a quiver high up on the right side of the patient's chest (Fig. 7.12).

5 Suction out. The suction tubing is also fixed next to the irrigation tubing over the left side of the patient's chest. The suction apparatus in our theatre is attached to the diathermy machine and the tubing therefore passes from the patient's left towards that machine. It is important that there is no coil of suction tubing on the floor which may be trod on by the surgeon causing suction to cease.

6 The camera. This is passed on to the operating table either in a sterile cover or having been sterilized in suitable fluid (for example: glutaraldehyde). The camera is placed between the patient's thighs and the lead passes up the left side of the patient's trunk towards the camera unit near the patient's left shoulder.

7 Light lead. The laparoscopic connection end of this is laid over the patient's thighs and passed alongside the camera lead towards the light unit near the patient's left shoulder.

8 Fixed retractors. If these are used they are fixed to the table at this stage. The one on the right is fixed to the table opposite the patient's iliac crest. It is used to hold the grasping forceps for the fundus and these are placed in position parallel with the patient's right flank. We also use a fixed retractor for the camera and this is placed in position on a level with the patient's left iliac crest.

9 Diathermy leads. Finally the diathermy lead or leads for attachment to the scissors and diathermy hook are passed out over the top of the other tubing from a point over the left side of the patient's chest. The leads are connected to the instruments which are placed in a sheath on the right side of the patient's chest.

Testing routines

Before any surgery is commenced the insufflator circuits are tested for leaks. We do this by connecting the gas in and vent out tubing together (using a plastic tube). The vent return is clamped off and the insufflator switched on. The circuit is pressurized and flow should rapidly cease. If flow continues there is a leak somewhere and this must be found and corrected before the operation proceeds.

If the operation is undertaken with a leak in the circuit there are two dangers.

1 The abdominal pressure is not correctly maintained.

2 When the exhaust gas circuit is switched on external air can be sucked into the circuit. This can produce a danger of an intraperitoneal explosion and in some cases can also lead to dangerous over-distension of the abdomen.

The Verres needle is also checked for adequate flow and that there are no leaks in the Verres needle circuit. With the tap fully open gas should flow freely, at zero pressure. If the tap is closed, flow should cease and the pressure indicator rise and alarm. If there is a leak in the Verres needle circuit, flow will be seen to occur even if the needle is blocked off. This would be misleading and dangerous during the initial critical stages of inducing the pneumoperitoneum when the surgeon relies on lack of flow to indicate incorrect positioning in the peritoneum.

The operation

Inserting the operative ports
The operative ports (cannulae) may be inserted in a variety of orders and positions. We will describe our usual practice here. Insertion of ports in the presence of adhesions is dealt with on p. 5 and 116–18.

First port (laparoscope) (Fig. 7.13)
This is a 10 mm port inserted through the umbilical incision. We prefer to use a guarded port (see p. 4). With the abdomen distended with at least 3 litres of gas, a trocar is placed in the cannula and using a rotatory movement introduced at a slight angle towards the pelvic cavity. A gas line is connected to this port. It is advisable to lift the abdominal wall anteriorly as for insertion of the Verres needle and to proceed slowly and carefully, especially when using an unguarded port. At this stage the theatre lights are dimmed. The camera is then inserted and the initial laparoscopy carried out (see p. 40).

Dangers
1 The trocar may penetrate bowel (especially when held by adhesions), the bladder, the bowel mesentery, retroperitoneal tissues or great vessels. The cannula may strike the posterior retroperitoneal

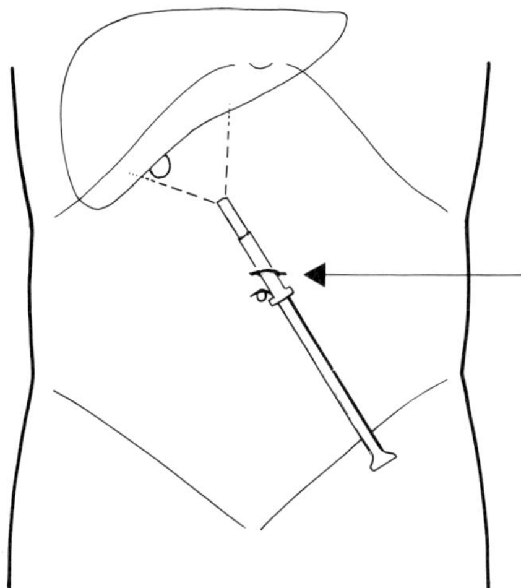

Fig. 7.13 The first port is situated above, below or through the umbilicus.

structures over the lower lumbar spine (this is very close in a thin subject, see Fig. 1.5). Look for these injuries as soon as the laparoscope is inserted. Hints on dealing with such injuries are given in Chapter 9, p. 112–14.

2 Subcutaneous or extraperitoneal cannulation. Even though a pneumoperitoneum has been successfully produced occasionally the cannula will only penetrate the subcutaneous or more frequently the extraperitoneal tissues. This is particularly a problem in obese subjects. Strands of areolar tissue and lobules of fat are seen with no view of the bowel. Inspect the area towards the abdominal cavity perpendicular to the anterior abdominal wall. You may be able to see a thinner area of peritoneum and having ascertained the direction, pass the trocar through it.

Hints

Do not turn the gas flow on to this port too soon. Pressure will probably be maintained until a second port is in place, and the cold gas will cool the laparoscope causing fogging.

Second port (left hand instruments) (Fig. 7.14)
We next place a 5 mm cannula in the right subcostal region. The gallbladder is visualized and the port placed close to and slightly lateral to the fundus of the gallbladder usually in the midclavicular

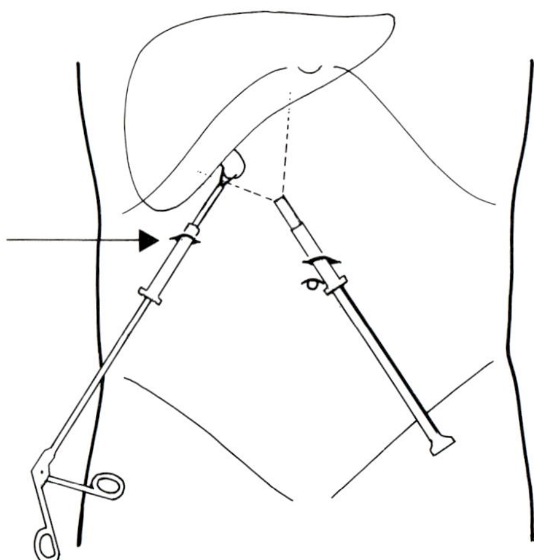

Fig. 7.14 The second, on the right side, subcostal port is situated in the midclavicular line. A grasper holds up the gallbladder.

line. Aim it towards the gallbladder. Make sure it is not in the direct line of view from the laparoscope to Calot's triangle.

Dangers
This port should be placed under direct vision and penetration of organs should not be a problem. Occasionally, a vessel may be punctured. This can be avoided by transilluminating the abdominal wall from within with the theatre lights turned down. Vessels can be seen and avoided.

Third port (for retraction of gallbladder fundus) (Fig. 7.15)
We next place another 5 mm cannula laterally in the anterior axillary line. This is again done under direct vision and the point to penetrate is visualized internally by dimpling the abdominal wall with a finger. Aim the port towards the fundus of the gallbladder.

Dangers
If this port is placed too far laterally there will be insufficient room to allow the grasper tips to be manoeuvred anteriorly as the handles will impinge on the patient's iliac crest.

Fourth port (right hand instruments) (Fig. 7.16)
This is a 10 mm cannula situated in the epigastrium usually just

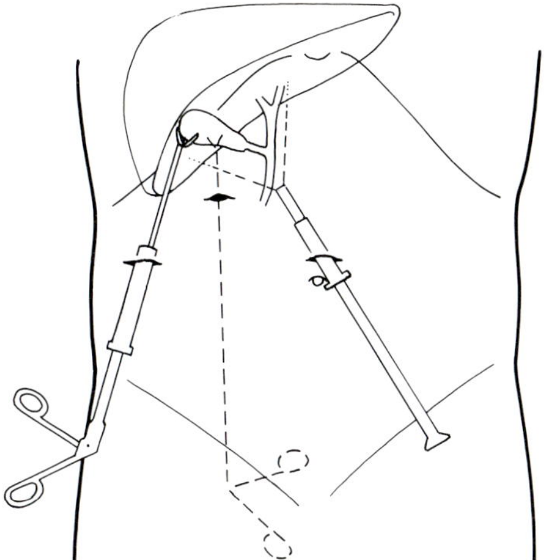

Fig. 7.15 The third port is situated, on the right side, laterally in the anterior axillary line and takes over retraction of the gallbladder fundus.

below the xiphisternum. Again, the insertion is done under direct vision. The initial penetration should be through the linea alba and the cannula is then moved to the right to come out at the angle between the anterior abdominal wall and the insertion of the right leaf of the falciform ligament (Fig. 7.17).

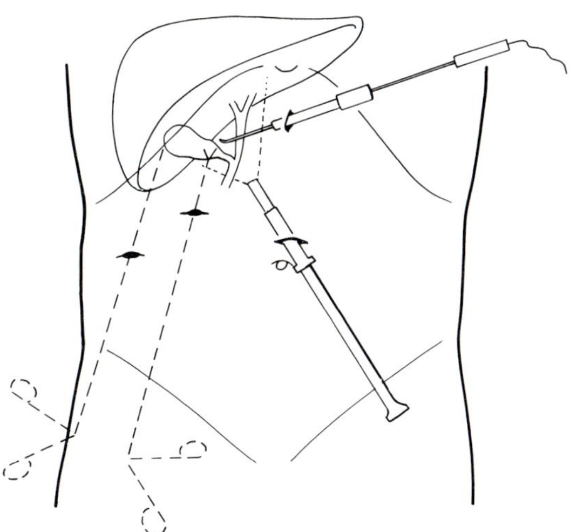

Fig. 7.16 The fourth port is situated in the epigastrium just below the xiphisternum and is the main instrumentation port.

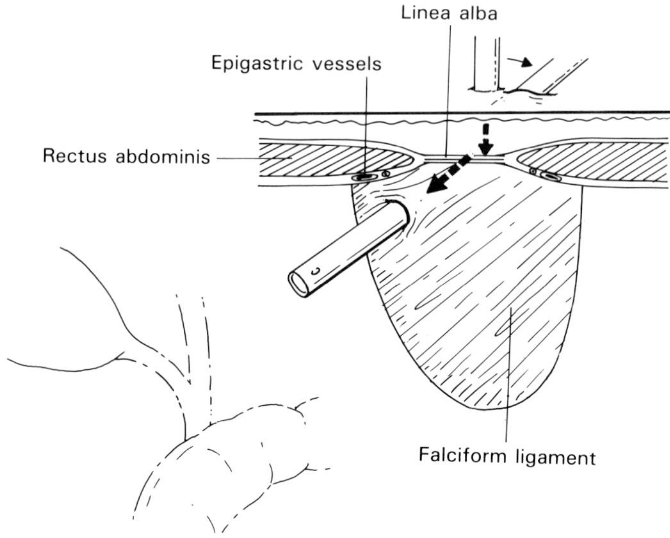

Fig. 7.17 We pass the epigastric cannula vertically through the linea alba and then turn to the right through the origin of the falciform ligament.

Dangers

If the port is put in obliquely, the trocar point can cut the superior epigastric artery which causes troublesome bleeding (see p. 112). A summary of the port positions are shown in Fig. 7.18.

An initial laparoscopy is then carried out as described on pp. 40–1.

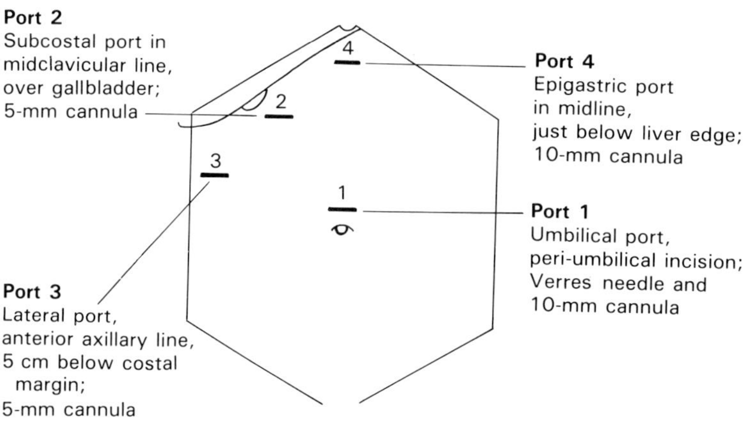

Fig. 7.18 Summary of the operating ports.

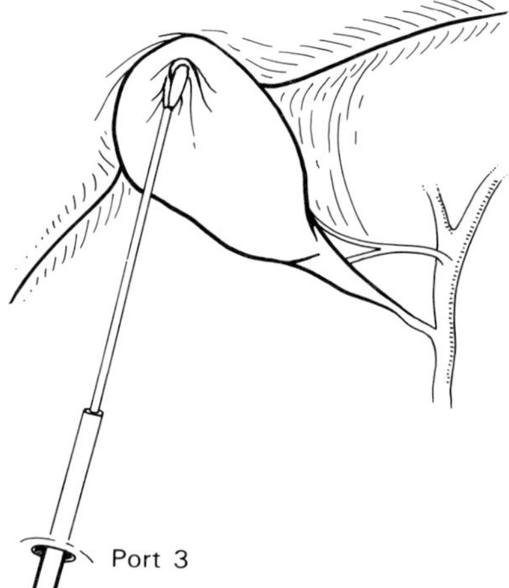

Fig. 7.19 The fundus of the gallbladder is pushed cranially and laterally by a grasper in port 3 in order to display Calot's triangle.

Exposure of Calot's triangle (e.g. cystic duct, artery and common bile duct)

The fundus of the gallbladder is pushed up and to the right over the liver using a grasping forceps in port 3. It is helpful to rotate the patient's foot down and rolled to the left so that the stomach, colon, and small bowel fall away from the operative site.

Retraction of the gallbladder

Technique
Calot's triangle is displayed by pushing the fundus of the gallbladder upwards and laterally (Fig. 7.19). Further retraction is produced by the graspers on the gallbladder neck.

Dangers
The graspers may tear the serosa or even the full thickness of the gallbladder wall.

Hints
1 If the gallbladder is very tense, empty it first either by inserting an aspirating needle or one of the 5 mm ports directly into the fundus of the gallbladder. The contents can then be aspirated and the gallbladder wall becomes easier to grasp. Where a trocar has been

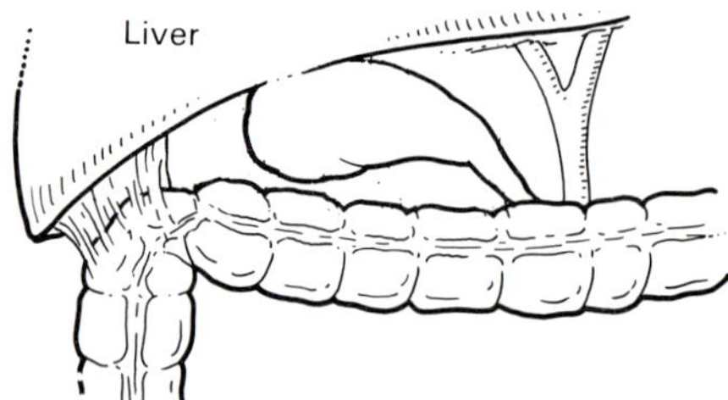

Fig. 7.20 Adhesions between the colon and the liver laterally can prevent visualization of the cystic duct.

inserted, the hole can be kept closed with the graspers used for retracting the fundus. Alternatively the hole can be closed with a preformed catgut loop.

2 Occasionally the gallbladder and liver are held to the parietal peritoneum by adhesions which must be divided to allow full retraction.

Adhesions to the gallbladder

These must be taken down in order to expose the lower end of the gallbladder and the cystic duct (Fig. 7.20). Adhesions between the colon and the under-surface of the liver should also be divided as these hold the colon up over the relevant anatomy. Occasionally there are also adhesions holding the left lobe over Calot's triangle. These should also be divided.

Technique
Light adhesions can be pulled down by blunt dissection. Firm adhesions should be divided with scissors or diathermy keeping close to the gallbladder.

Dangers
1 The serosa is stripped off the gallbladder exposing the mucosa which may rupture later in the operation.
2 Vessels in the adhesions are divided and these continue bleeding out of sight once they have retracted caudally.

Hints
1 Use graspers in your left hand (port 2) to put gentle traction on the adhesions; then divide them close to their origin on the gallbladder. If they look as though they contain vessels, diathermy them first.

2 Do not lose sight of the adhesion until you are sure it is not bleeding.

3 Separation of adherent colon and duodenum (see p. 119).

4 The initial stage of exposing Calot's triangle can be tedious and difficult but patience is essential if crippling injury to the bile duct is to be avoided.

Defining the cystic duct

Technique
Once the adhesions and neighbouring organs have been separated from the gallbladder, the area of the cystic duct becomes visible. The peritoneum over Calot's triangle needs to be opened either with a diathermy hook or scissors or possibly by blunt dissection. We favour careful use of the diathermy hook. Once the peritoneum has been divided, push it medially and laterally and the cystic duct and artery will gradually become apparent.

When the cystic duct is seen, divide the strands on and around it using the 'hook, look, cook' technique as described on p. 43. This allows the duct to straighten out. Manoeuvre the duct into a suitable position for dissection using graspers attached to the neck of the gallbladder and held in the left hand through port 2. As strands are divided, the duct gradually straightens. Keep very close to its wall and go round it posteriorly with curved dissecting forceps. It is often easier to find the posterior layer than the anterior wall of the duct. Encircle the duct where it is easy to do so and then extend the separation of the duct medially and laterally so that a suitable length is exposed. Make quite certain this duct is in continuity with the neck of the gallbladder. If there is any doubt, go further up towards the gallbladder before dissecting any further.

Dangers
Beware of abnormal anatomy, e.g. a posterior duct which may be a continuation of a right hepatic duct or the common bile duct itself. Again, if in doubt, move further up the neck of the gallbladder.

Hints
If the isolation of the duct is proving difficult, go laterally and dissect posteriorly at the level of Hartmann's pouch keeping close to the

gallbladder wall. Once a plane has been found around the gallbladder at this relatively safe level, you can then move medially down the gallbladder wall until you encounter the cystic duct.

Cholangiogram

We routinely perform a cholangiogram at this stage in order to be quite certain that our interpretation of the anatomy is correct. We use the technique described by Dr J. Petelin of Kansas and find it both easy and satisfactory as do our various trainees. The technique should be practised in a simulator to obtain confidence before attempting it in a patient.

Techniques

PETELIN TECHNIQUE

Having thoroughly cleaned and straightened the cystic duct, two clips are applied close to the neck of the gallbladder. The duct is incised on its cranial margin using scissors through the epigastric port (number 4). Care is taken not to transect the whole duct. The opening is enlarged until bile is seen to flow from it. This can be done with microscissors if necessary.

We use a subclavian vein cannulation set, comprising a 16 gauge round-ended intravenous catheter and needle, passed through a 13 gauge cannula.

An intravenous needle and cannula is placed slightly medial and cranial to port 2 and under direct vision enters the peritoneal cavity. It should not be in the line of view between the laparoscope and Calot's triangle. The needle is withdrawn. The intravenous catheter is then passed through the sheath and picked up with curved dissecting forceps in the peritoneal cavity. This is best performed while only a small length of cannula has been pushed through, since it is steadied by the abdominal wall while the correct grip is obtained. The angle at which the cannula is picked up is critical and it should be in line with the curve of the forceps at about 135° to the shaft of the instrument. About 1.5–2 cm of the catheter protrudes from the tip of the forceps.

The catheter is then carried down towards the cystic duct and the laparoscope zoomed in on this part of the anatomy. The cystic duct is manoeuvred into a satisfactory position using the forceps attached

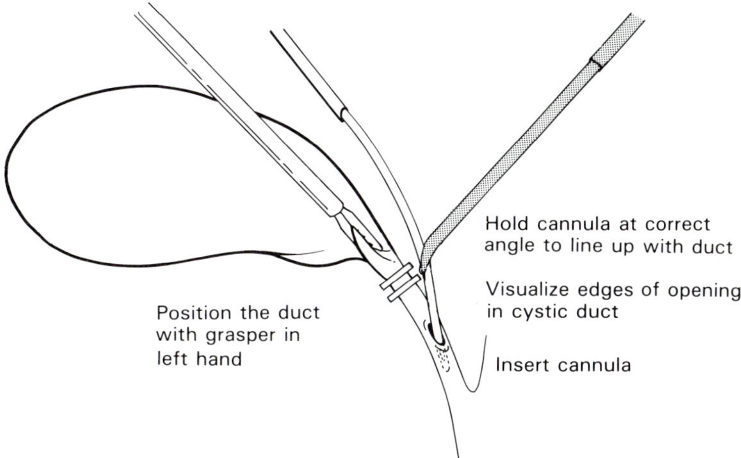

Fig. 7.21 Insertion of the cholangiogram catheter into the cystic duct. The duct is positioned by the grasper in the subcostal port. The cannula is held by the epigastric port grasper.

to the neck of the gallbladder with the left hand. Lateral traction is also maintained on the cystic duct to keep it straight (Fig. 7.21). It is usually easy to insert the catheter into the lumen of the cystic duct and push it medially.

Once the cannula is satisfactorily in position, the dissecting forceps is removed and replaced with a clip applicator. One clip is applied to the cystic duct around the catheter. A 20 cm³ syringe containing saline is attached to the catheter and saline injected by the surgeon. As this is performed, the clip is gradually closed until resistance to the flow of saline is felt. At this point pressure on the clip is released. The clip is now sufficiently closed to hold the catheter in position but not to obstruct the flow.

The metal graspers in ports 2 and 4 are now withdrawn and the grasper in port 3 holding the fundus is released preventing traction on the gallbladder and cystic duct from kinking the common bile duct (Fig. 7.22).

Any metal ports are lined up in a craniocaudal direction so that they do not obscure the X-ray picture. We stick them down with adhesive tape. The laparoscope is removed and the insufflator turned off. There is no need to deflate the abdomen. The gas input, gas exhaust and return tubes should be disconnected so that intraperitoneal fluid does not run back into the insufflator during the X-ray. The

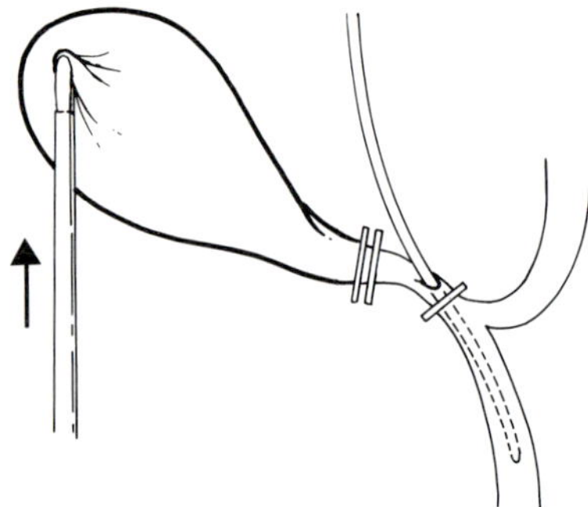

Fig. 7.22 Traction on the gallbladder can kink the biliary tree and prevent filling of the upper hepatic ducts on a cholangiogram.

table is levelled out and may be rolled slightly to the patient's right. The X-ray apparatus is lined up. We usually take two films, one after injecting $10\,cm^3$ of Urograffin 150 (Schering Ltd) and another after injecting another $10\,cm^3$.

REDDICK–OLSEN CHOLANGIOGRAM CLAMP

An alternative technique is to use the Reddick–Olsen cholangiogram clamp manufactured by Storz. This inserts the catheter into the duct and then holds it in place with one instrument. We have not found the additional expense of this instrument to be necessary. The dexterity acquired by repeated insertion of catheters into the cystic duct has proved useful when removing stones from the common bile duct.

Dangers

The cystic duct may be divided completely and be difficult to retrieve.

There may be a stone in the distal end of the cystic duct which either obstructs the passage of the catheter or is pushed into the common bile duct by the catheter.

No image of the left and right hepatic ducts is produced because traction on the cystic duct is causing an acute kink in the common bile duct at the entry of the cystic duct. This is due to failure to release the traction on the fundus of the gallbladder.

Hints

1 Do not be deterred by initial difficulties with the technique. Everybody experiences these and persistence will be rewarded as confidence grows.

2 Practice in a simulator.

3 If the lumen of the cystic duct is clearly smaller than the catheter then we would not persist with the cholangiogram. This occurs in 5–10% of cases. In such cases it is also very unlikely that a stone has passed into the common bile duct or that the duct you are cannulating is either the right hepatic or the common bile duct. Before making this decision it is, however, essential to have assessed the internal diameter of the duct correctly and not to be misled by having made too small an opening in the duct.

4 If a cholangiogram is being performed it is advisable not to divide the cystic artery until the cholangiogram is completed. Should the cystic duct part, the artery will hold the gallbladder in towards the porta hepatis and this makes it easier to retrieve the end of the cystic duct. Once the artery has been divided it is much more difficult to find structures medially.

If the X-ray shows stones in the biliary tree then proceed as on pp. 101–7.

Removing the catheter

Technique
If the anatomy is confirmed when the X-ray is available, the cystic duct clip is removed by grasping its angle and pulling it off the duct in the line of the clip. The catheter is then removed. The cystic duct is doubly clipped proximally and divided.

The cystic artery

Technique
Initially, we tried to dissect out the cystic artery early in the operation but more recently we have been content to find and isolate it after the cystic duct has been divided. It usually lies directly behind the cystic duct and is much easier to visualize once the duct is out of the way. Where possible the main stem is isolated and doubly clipped and divided. In many cases, however, the anterior and posterior cystic artery have to be divided separately.

Dangers
Some of these have been dealt with under the section on abnormal

anatomy. The main danger is cutting an uncontrolled posterior cystic artery.

If excessive traction is put on the gallbladder after the cystic duct has been divided and before the cystic artery has been isolated, the artery may tear and the area be obscured by haemorrhage. As in all dissections in this operation, gentleness and patience are keywords.

If the artery is easily visible before division of the cystic duct then it may with benefit be clipped at that time, but not divided.

It is safer to clip the main cystic artery but small branches can be diathermied.

Freeing the gallbladder from its bed

Once the cystic duct and all the cystic arterial branches have been divided, the gallbladder lifts away from its bed exposing the connective tissue between it and the liver. Occasionally this is in the form of a mesentery which is easy to divide but all variations of attachment up to a complete intrahepatic gallbladder may be encountered.

Technique

Using the graspers in the left hand, the gallbladder is held close to the area to be dissected and traction is maintained to expose the areolar or fibrous tissue to be divided. This is then divided with the preferred instrument. We use the diathermy hook or scissors medially and the contact tip laser laterally.

As the separation continues, it becomes difficult to maintain adequate traction with the left-handed graspers and these must be repositioned on the gallbladder at regular intervals.

Dangers

Hepatic veins may be encountered if the dissection strays too far into the liver. This can produce troublesome haemorrhage (see pp. 115–16). If the dissection is carried too close to the gallbladder it may be perforated with leakage of bile and stones. This is not a disaster but is best avoided as it can be troublesome to retrieve lost stones and the gallbladder may spill more stones as it is being extracted from the abdomen.

Hints

1 The critical manoeuvre is to keep in the right layer and stretch the

tissues in this layer with accurately placed traction. As you approach the fundus of the gallbladder, move the position of the grasper attached to the fundus through port 3, keeping it close to the area being dissected.

2 The most difficult part of the dissection occurs over the back of the fundus of the gallbladder as the dissection is nearing its end. Do not hurry this.

The gallbladder bed

Once the gallbladder has been freed it should be held in a grasper and placed above the liver out of the way and attention paid to haemostasis in the gallbladder bed.

Technique

A grasper in the lateral port (number 3) can be used to hold up the liver and diathermy graspers or a ball-point diathermy can be inserted through the epigastric port (number 4). Sometimes it is beneficial to reverse the position of these instruments. Where there is troublesome venous bleeding a blunt diathermy instrument placed lightly in contact with the tissues around the bleeding area is often the most effective way of achieving haemostasis. Small vessels at the lateral edge of the gallbladder bed should also be diathermied. At this stage there should rarely be any bleeding in the more medial area of the gallbladder bed.

Dangers

Excessive pressure on the diathermy may cause a burn which penetrates deeper into the gallbladder bed opening up larger vessels.

Hints

1 Brush the diathermy instrument lightly over the bleeding surface. This produces a coagulum without penetrating deep into the liver.

2 A bare fibre laser or one with a ball sapphire tip, can also be useful for producing haemostasis at this time (see Fig. 4.12, p. 46).

Inserting a drain

The use of drains after cholecystectomy has always been contentious. We do not routinely drain an open cholecystectomy but we do feel this is beneficial in a laparoscopic procedure and use a drain routinely. We believe that this has the following advantages.

1 The removal of remaining intraperitoneal gas.
2 Removal of remaining intraperitoneal fluid and blood. In common with others we have formed the impression that this factor together with removal of intraperitoneal gas decreases postoperative abdominal and shoulder pain.
3 The presence of a drain has allowed the early detection of intraperitoneal bleeding.

The removal of residual gas and fluid occurs as soon as muscular tone returns to the abdominal wall and we routinely remove the drain 2 hours postoperatively.

Technique

A 14 gauge drain normally used with a suction apparatus is passed in through port 3 and grasped with forceps placed in port 2 or 4. It is easily positioned in the subhepatic area. It is then held internally and the cannula in port 3 is removed over the top of the drain. The drain is then sutured in position. The suture also prevents further leakage of gas. The drain is clamped until the pneumoperitoneum is no longer required.

Dangers

We have not encountered any disadvantages to inserting a drain, though it does sometimes cause pain which is relieved when it is removed.

Haemostasis

Before removing the gallbladder and the laparoscopic instruments, a thorough check is made of the abdominal cavity including the following.
1 The gallbladder bed.
2 The porta hepatis.
3 Adhesions divided from the gallbladder and omentum.
4 Elsewhere in the abdomen.

Any areas with clot should be thoroughly washed and bleeding points picked up and controlled. As in all forms of abdominal surgery, time spent at this stage can markedly diminish postoperative problems.

Peritoneal toilet

Technique

The peritoneal cavity is washed out with heparinized saline and all clot and bile removed until the washout effluent is clear. This also confirms that there is no continued bleeding. Some clear fluid may then be left in the abdomen and allowed to drain out through the drain in the first postoperative hours.

Extracting the gallbladder

Having completed peritoneal toilet and established haemostasis, the gallbladder can now be removed. This phase of the operation should not be hurried. Rupture of the gallbladder and spillage of stones through excessive haste can markedly prolong an operation which had appeared to be almost over.

The gallbladder can be extracted either via the umbilical port or the epigastric port. We prefer the latter.

The advantages of the umbilical port are that the scar remains hidden even if it is extended. The disadvantages are that the camera port has to be changed to the epigastrium and this makes hand/eye coordination much more difficult for the surgeon. In addition, if the gallbladder does drop stones these tend to disappear in loops of bowel. Finally an extended incision in the umbilical area is more likely to be followed by late herniation.

The advantages of the epigastric port are that normal vision and hand/eye coordination is maintained. If stones do fall from the gallbladder, they drop onto the liver and can often easily be extracted. The disadvantages are that the view may be somewhat obscured by the falciform ligament though this is not a serious disadvantage in our experience. If the scar has to be enlarged to remove the gallbladder it is more visible than an umbilical scar.

Technique

The gallbladder is manoeuvred into position just below the liver where it can be easily seen through the laparoscope. A large 10 mm grasping forceps or claw forceps is placed through the 10 mm cannula in the extraction port and the neck of the gallbladder is grasped in the region of the previously applied cystic duct clips. The neck of the gallbladder is then gently manoeuvred into the port and the port slowly extracted from the abdomen. The theatre lights are turned on and the neck of the gallbladder is held with haemostats as it appears through the skin. The gallbladder is then opened externally and a sucker inserted and the bile emptied. Stones may be extracted using Desjardin's forceps. Large stones can be crushed or broken up. A view of the outside wall of the gallbladder is maintained through the laparoscope in the abdomen to make sure there are no signs of rupture. If there are such signs then it is wiser to extend the extraction port and remove the gallbladder easily through it. We have found no disadvantages in such an extended inclusion as far as postoperative recovery is concerned.

Dangers
Excessive traction on the gallbladder may result in rupture and loss of stones.

Hints
1 It is important to grasp the clips on the cystic duct obliquely as clips at right angle to the cannula can obstruct it.
2 Where there is already a hole in the gallbladder or where rupture seems likely, it can be useful to extract the gallbladder within a bag. This may be either a small plastic bag, a condom, or a specially designed laparoscopic bag (Espiner bag). The technique of using this bag is described below.
3 If the insufflating gas was attached to the extraction port, move it to one of the remaining ports.
4 For difficulties in extraction see p. 128.

Use of a bag for extraction
See Fig. 7.23.

Technique
The 'tail' attached to the bag is pulled through a reducing sleeve. Grasping forceps are passed down the reducing sleeve and the apex of the bag held in them. The bag is then pushed down through a 10 mm port (we use the epigastric one) and the reducing sleeve placed in position. The bag is completely placed within the abdomen and its neck opened. The gallbladder is then placed within the bag and the cystic duct found and held with the graspers. The cystic duct

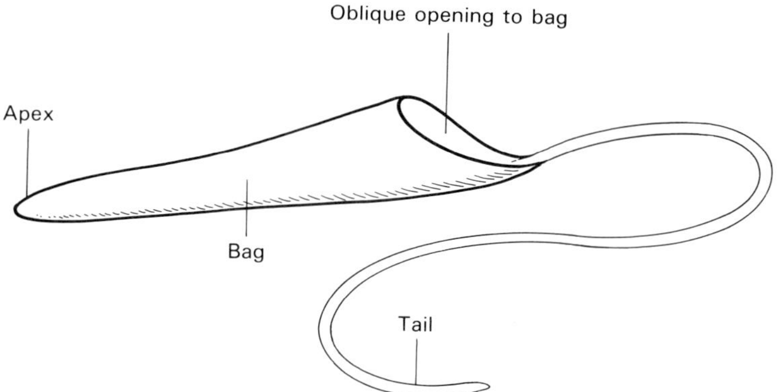

Fig. 7.23 The Espiner bag is made of hot air balloon fabric and can be autoclaved. The tail is used to pull it back through the extraction port.

is positioned at the opening of the exit cannula. The tail of the bag is then drawn out of the cannula and the cannula and the bag extracted. The oblique design of the neck means the bag closes off as it is withdrawn into the port.

Enlarging the exit port

Technique

We have developed a technique for enlarging the exit port safely. The gallbladder will have been pulled up into the exit wound already. The skin is first incised with a sharp pointed knife beside the gallbladder. A grooved director is then passed into the wound and seen to emerge within the abdomen through the laparoscope. This is positioned craniocaudally so that the groove faces the linea alba in the midline. A knife with a number 11 blade is then slid down the grooved director with the sharp edge of the knife towards the linea alba (Fig. 7.24). The linea alba is thus incised in the midline and the port enlarged. If this technique is carried out correctly there should be no bleeding and even a very large gallbladder can be extracted easily.

The linea alba is then sutured using polyglactin on a J-shaped needle as below.

Closing the linea alba

If the port has not been enlarged we have not found it necessary to close the linea alba though some surgeons do undertake this. We always close the fascial layer if the exit has been enlarged.

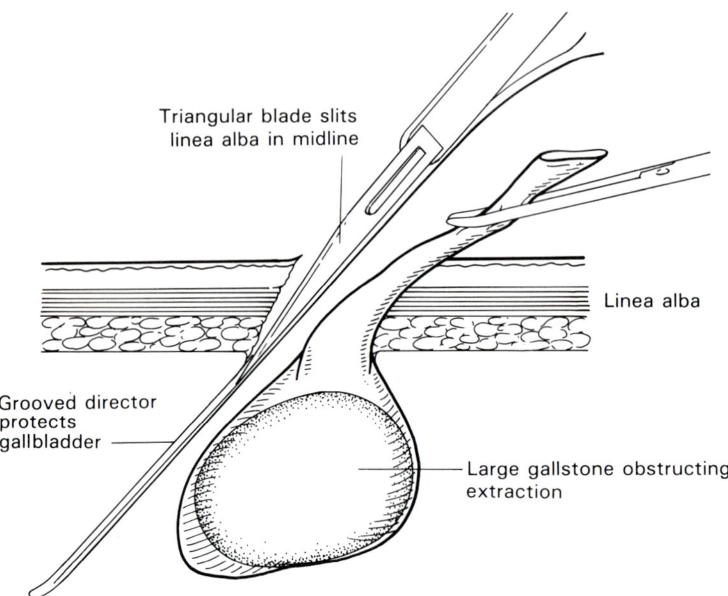

Fig. 7.24 A grooved director is used to protect the gallbladder while enlarging the incision in the linea alba.

Technique

The wound is spread with two Langenbeck retractors. A J-shaped needle is inserted in the wound moving the point from within the abdomen towards the outside. A similar manoeuvre is carried out on the opposite side of the fascia. Before this is tied, a second suture may be inserted. Both are then tied and the closure is tested with a finger. The light of the laparoscope may be positioned underneath the incision producing useful illumination.

Closing the skin

Technique

The skin may be closed with sutures, clips or staples. We prefer subcuticular polyglactin sutures as these are absorbable and give a very good cosmetic result.

Problems

With very early discharge of patients, sutures which have to be removed are an added complication. It is sometimes difficult to insert sutures in the incisions for 5 mm ports and these can be advantageously closed with adhesive strips.

If metal clips or staples are used these can be removed after 24 hours.

As mentioned above, we remove our drain after 2 hours. If we are suspicious of a bile leak or other problem the drain may be left longer.

8: Stones in the hepatic and common bile ducts

The problem
Methods of management
   Stones found before operation
   Stones found during operation
Laparoscopic techniques for bile duct
    exploration
   Exploration under X-ray control

Exploration through a
   choledochotomy
Exploration using a flexible
   choledochoscope
Laparoscopic lithotripsy of
   common duct stones

The problem

Patients may be found to have stones in the biliary tract before or during cholecystectomy. These must either be passed or removed before treatment is complete. Experience with laparoscopic surgery for stones in the hepatic and common bile ducts is still limited.

Stones can be suspected to be present in the common duct if:

1 The patient remains jaundiced.

2 There has been a recent episode of jaundice or pancreatitis.

3 The bilirubin or alkaline phosphatase were raised during a recent acute attack of pain.

4 The common duct is dilated on ultrasound (more than 10 mm diameter).

Because the presence of common duct stones cannot be accurately predicted before laparoscopic operation, all patients must be warned of the possibility of discovering stones in the duct and told the full plan of action if these are found. This explanation must include the possibility of postoperative endoscopic exploration of the common duct and also the small possibility of late open exploration of the duct. We present our patients with a sheet containing this information (see Appendix).

Methods of management

Possible techniques for clearing stones from the biliary tract include:

1 Endoscopic sphincterotomy and retrograde exploration of the common bile duct through the duodenum.

2 Open exploration of the common duct.

3 Laparoscopic exploration of the common duct by one of the methods described below.

Stones found before operation

We would at present try to carry out a precholecystectomy endoscopic sphincterotomy. In 85% of patients, common duct stones can be removed by this technique. If this fails then the options are open cholecystectomy and exploration of the common bile duct (especially if the stones are larger than 10 mm diameter) or laparoscopic exploration of the common duct (see below). We prefer the latter but the choice will depend on the surgeon's experience and the size and expected difficulty of removing the common duct stones.

Stones found during operation

If operative cholangiography is carried out routinely, a percentage (4% in our series) of patients will be found to have common duct stones during the operation which were unexpected, with no pre-operative history of jaundice or pancreatitis. A decision will then have to be made at operation, as to how to proceed. The options are:

1 Complete the cholecystectomy leaving the stones in the duct and arrange an endoscopic sphincterotomy and stone removal postoperatively. If this fails, the patient will need an open exploration of the duct.

2 Attempt removal of the stones laparoscopically. If successful, much has been gained. If this fails then an endoscopic retrograde cholangiopancreatogram (ERCP) can still be arranged, and again a final resort to open exploration on a separate occasion is still a possibility.

Laparoscopic techniques for bile duct exploration

Several individual techniques may be made use of including:

1 Exploration of the common bile duct under X-ray control only.

2 Exploration of the common bile duct under direct vision using a choledochoscope.

These may be combined with:

3 Balloon dilatation of the cystic duct and sphincter of Oddi.

4 Balloon extraction of stones via the cystic duct.

5 Dormia basket extraction of stones via the cystic duct.

6 Intra-operative lithotripsy of cystic duct stones with laser, electro-static, ultrasound or mechanical lithotripsy and extraction of fragments.

7 Extraction of stones via direct incision in the supraduodenal common bile duct.

In our experience laparoscopic exploration of the common bile duct is worthwhile even if a choledochoscope is not available. An

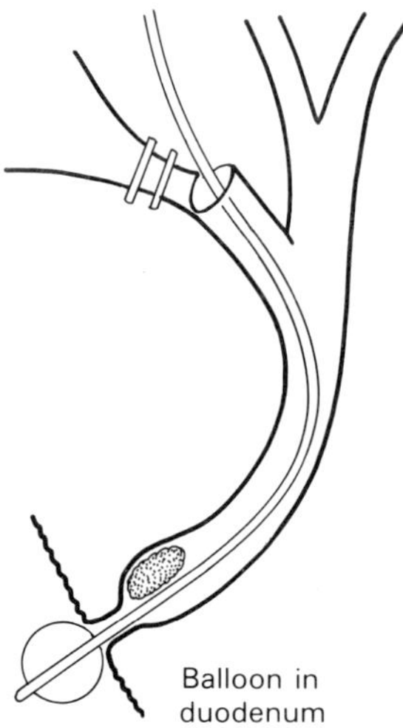

Fig. 8.1 Using a balloon to find the sphincter of Oddi. The inflated balloon is passed into the duodenum and pulled back against the sphincter.

X-ray image intensifier would make the task easier but the duct can sometimes be cleared without this equipment. We do not have one available in theatre.

Exploration under X-ray control

This method is suitable for stones of less than 10 mm in diameter. Very little additional equipment is necessary (a Dormia basket, see pp. 26–7, and a 4 gauge Fogarty embolectomy catheter), but it can take a long time due to the need for repeated check X-rays.

A peroperative cholangiogram is carried out as on p. 88. The position of the stones in the common bile duct is noted. Fortunately these are frequently in the lower part of the duct. The clip securing the cholangiogram catheter in the cystic duct is removed and the catheter extracted. It is replaced with a 4 French gauge Fogarty balloon which is passed down the Intracath cannula used for the cholangiogram catheter. It is passed right down the duct into the duodenum. The balloon is inflated and this can be seen laparoscopically causing a bulge in the duodenal wall. The catheter is then retracted until it impacts on the sphincter of Oddi (Fig. 8.1). The position of the catheter is noted either by marks on its surface or by holding it in a set position with grasping forceps. The balloon is deflated and the catheter withdrawn 5–10 mm. Easy inflation of

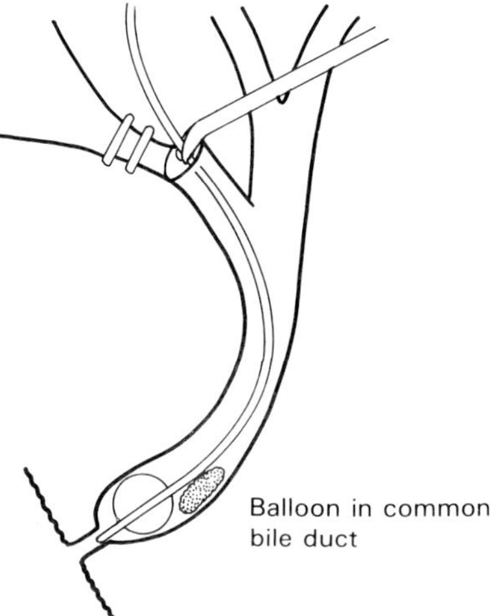

Fig. 8.2 The balloon is deflated, withdrawn and reinflated in the common bile duct.

the balloon indicates that it is now back in the common bile duct (Fig. 8.2). It is passed a little distally until dilatation of the balloon is difficult. At this point it is situated in the sphincter (Fig. 8.3). The sphincter is dilated by blowing up the balloon. The balloon is deflated and the catheter is withdrawn into the cystic duct (Fig. 8.4b). The cystic duct is similarly dilated by inflating the balloon until the

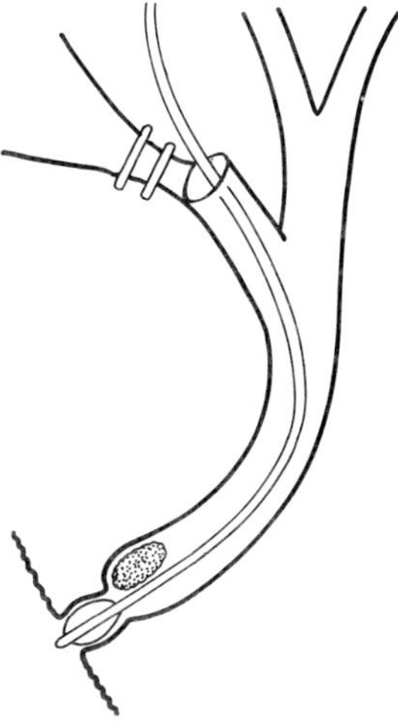

Fig. 8.3 Having noted the two previous positions, the balloon can be placed in the sphincter itself.

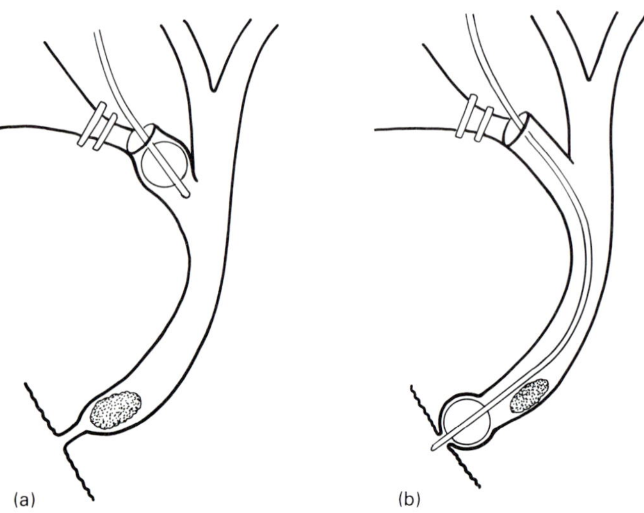

Fig. 8.4 (a) Dilating the cystic duct with the balloon. (b) Dilating the sphincter of Oddi with the balloon.

inflated balloon can be withdrawn from the cystic duct (Fig. 8.4a). The Fogarty catheter is then removed.

A Dormia basket is now pressed through the catheter sheath and manoeuvred down the cystic duct noting each centimetre that is passed. It is usually about 5 cm to the sphincter. The position can be checked by passing the Dormia basket into the duodenum and opening the basket. It can then be pulled back so that it impacts on the sphincter of Oddi and the position noted. The basket is collapsed and the instrument withdrawn into the common bile duct so as to position it at the site of the stone. Remember that the basket opens beyond the tip of the catheter and it may therefore be necessary to withdraw the catheter a little further to allow for this. Open the basket at the presumed site of the stone and close it again. If it closes completely the stone has not been caught. If it will not close completely the stone has been encountered (Fig. 8.5). Withdraw it carefully and slowly up the cystic duct. It may be necessary to incise the cystic duct to widen the opening and allow extraction of the stone. Reinsert the cholangiogram catheter, repeat the X-ray and remove further fragments as indicated, washing the duct out with saline between extractions. When the duct is finally clear, tie off the cystic duct. This usually requires a catgut loop as it is too large to be closed with a clip.

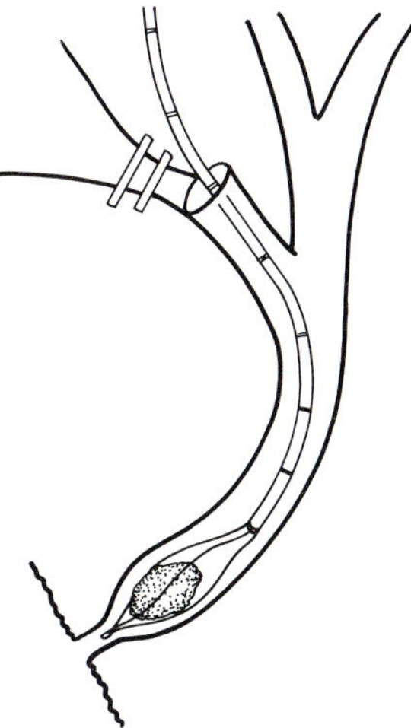

Fig. 8.5 Retrieving a stone from the lower end of the common bile duct with a Dormia basket.

Soft stones of more than 1 cm in diameter are sometimes broken up by the basket in which case the fragments can then be extracted as above. If a large stone cannot be broken up, explore the duct via a choledochotomy as below.

Exploration through a choledochotomy
Tie off or clip the cystic duct. Dissect the areolar tissue off the front wall of the common bile duct being careful not to damage the fine vessels on the front of the duct. Decide where a choledochotomy is to be made and seal off any visible surface vessels using point diathermy with the tip of the diathermy hook. Incise the front wall of the common bile duct. A contact laser is ideal for this and produces good haemostasis. If one is not available, micro-dissecting scissors should be used. Open the duct with forceps and extract the stone either with forceps, with a basket, or with a balloon.

Choose a T-tube of suitable size and trim it as for open duct exploration. Pass the whole T-tube through the epigastric 10 mm port so that it lies freely within the abdominal cavity. Pick up one limb of the T-tube with forceps situated in the epigastric port. Manoeuvre it into the distal common bile duct. Pushing that limb distally, manoeuvre the second limb into the duct proximally. The duct itself can be steadied with forceps through the subcostal port.

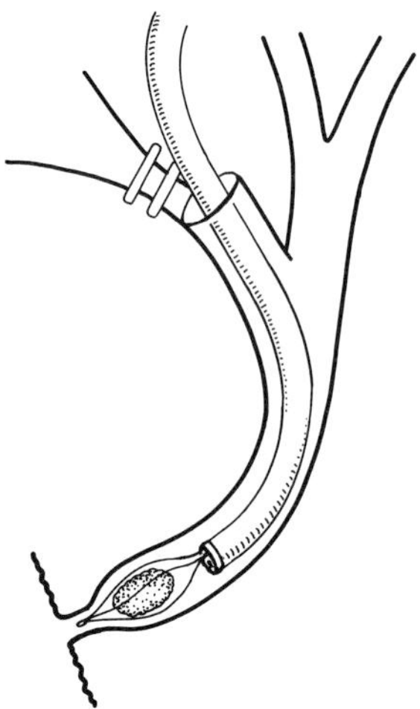

Fig. 8.6 Common bile duct stone retrieval using a choledochoscope.

Suture the duct walls together over the T-tube using interrupted 4/0 polyglactin or catgut.

At the end of the operation, grasp the long stem of the T-tube via the subcostal port and withdraw it and the port together preventing tension on the common duct end by holding the tube internally with forceps. Check that the inner end remains in position in the duct by viewing it through the laparoscope. Fix the T-tube in place using a skin suture. Position a drain as on pp. 93–4. The further management is as for open cholecystectomy and exploration of the common bile duct. We carry out a T-tube cholangiogram on the seventh postoperative day and remove the tube immediately if the X-ray is clear.

Exploration using a flexible choledochoscope (Petelin's method)
The cystic duct is cannulated with a flexible guide wire introduced through the subcostal port. Ureteric dilators are then passed down this guide wire and used to dilate the cystic duct up to the size of the available choledochoscope. Either a small flexible choledochoscope, ureteroscope, or even an intravascular scope may be suitable. It should have an operating channel through which a Dormia basket can be passed. The scope is introduced through the subcostal port and manoeuvred into the cystic duct with forceps through the epigastric port. It is passed down into the common bile duct and the stone visualized. A second camera and screen can be used for this purpose. A basket is passed down the operating channel and the

stone grasped and removed (Fig. 8.6). It can be useful to pass a
Fogarty catheter through a separate port down the cystic duct along-
side the choledochoscope and inflate the balloon beyond the stone.
The choledochoscope, stone and balloon are then removed together.
The duct can then be cleared under direct vision.

By retracting the cystic duct caudally it is sometimes possible to
manoeuvre the scope into the proximal hepatic ducts but a low
insertion of the cystic duct can make this impossible.

Laparoscopic lithotripsy of common duct stones
The apparatus to carry this out is expensive but if it is available,
stones can be shattered by probes passed either down the cystic duct
or directly through a choledochotomy. Energy is delivered direct to
the stone in the form of high frequency ultrasound, laser energy or
electrostatic shock waves and the stone shattered. Larger fragments
can then be removed, and the rest left to pass.

9: Dealing with operative difficulties

Technical problems
  Loss of vision
  Fogging of laparoscope
  Obesity
  Loss of pneumoperitoneum
Haemorrhage
  Bleeding from ports
  Retroperitoneal haematoma
  Major haemorrhage into the
    peritoneal cavity, origin unclear
  Major haemorrhage from hepatic
    or cystic arteries, or portal vein
  Haemorrhage from the gallbladder
    bed
Problems due to inflammation and
    fibrosis
  Peritoneal adhesions
  Adherent duodenum and colon
  Small shrunken gallbladder
  Empyema of the gallbladder
  Fibrosis around the portal triad
  Oedematous thickened gallbladder
    wall

Problems due to surgical trauma
  Verres needle or trocar injuries
  Damage to the bowel
  Damage to hepatic or common bile
    ducts
  Hole in the gallbladder
  Loss of stones in the peritoneum
  CO_2 embolism
  Loss of a needle in the peritoneal
    cavity
Anatomical and pathological
    difficulties
  Distended gallbladder
  Intrahepatic gallbladder
  Abnormal anatomy
  Stones in the cystic duct
  Stones in the common bile duct
  Short cystic duct
  Wide cystic duct
  Large stones
  Difficult extraction
Collapse of patient

Technical problems

Loss of vision

This may be complete, or more often, partial. Complete loss of vision is due to camera, light source, or electrical failure. If the problem cannot be corrected it may be necessary to open the patient.

Partial loss of vision

This is due to the following.

1 Electrical interference: check that the diathermy lead is not crossing the camera lead or that other machines are not causing the interference.

2 Poor connections: check that all the leads are pressed 'home' in their sockets.

3 Condensation: see fogging of the laparoscope below.

4 Fat or blood on the lenses: a dirty swab may deposit a film of fat on the camera or the eyepiece as it is wiped free of moisture. Keep all blood-stained or soiled swabs out of reach of the surgeon.

Fat on the distal end of the scope due to contact with the omentum is a more common problem. The laparoscope must be withdrawn and cleaned. It may be useful to replace it in the warming bath for a short period.

5 Smoke from the diathermy or laser. Smoke will diminish the transmission, reflection and reception of light. It can persist for a long time in the peritoneal cavity. A smoke extraction system is essential in our opinion. Make sure the smoke extraction system is switched on and working. The sucker can also be used to remove smoke but as it has no return system this is at the expense of loss of the pneumoperitoneum. Make sure the smoke extraction outlet is not via the laparoscope port or smoke will be continually drawn into view.

6 Loss of the pneumoperitoneum (see below p. 112).

7 A damaged light cable.

8 A cracked casing or lens in the laparoscope. Direct vision down the scope is also poor.

Fogging of laparoscope

The problem

This is commonly due to condensation on the internal end of the laparoscope when that instrument is colder than the peritoneal cavity. Causes include the following.

1 Insufficient pre-operative warming.

2 Cold gas blowing over the shaft of the instrument.

3 Condensation between the camera and the eyepiece.

4 Cold operating theatre environment.

Hints

1 The laparoscope should be warmed thoroughly before surgery begins. We use a bottle of sterile water warmed to 40° and kept warm in an electrically heated bath, adapted from a blood warming apparatus (see p. 13). It is important to insert the laparoscope at least 15 minutes before it is used. Otherwise, only the tip is warm and heat is transferred away from this to the colder part of the instrument.

2 Within the abdomen the laparoscope can be defogged by wiping it on a loop of small bowel or the liver. However this sometimes produces a film of fat over the lens. This is especially so if the omentum is touched. The end of the laparoscope can get quite hot so beware of wiping grease away in this manner.

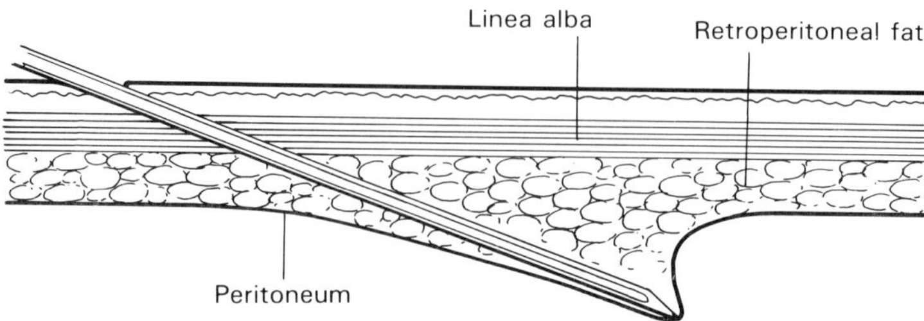

Fig. 9.1 Loose peritoneum may be pushed out in front of the needle or trocar.

3 Connect the gas inlet to a separate port to the one containing the laparoscope.

4 Consider raising the temperature of the operating theatre.

5 The other place condensation occurs is at the camera–laparoscope interface. Sterilization fluid may remain there and vaporize as the operation proceeds. Disconnect the camera and wipe both it and the laparoscope eyepiece dry.

6 A ventilated camera–laparoscope interface can prevent condensation here.

Obesity

As most of the excess fat in an obese patient is in the subcutaneous tissues it is often less difficult to remove the gallbladder laparoscopically than by open cholecystectomy.

Patients will often be willing to lose weight prior to surgery and this may be beneficial as far as their postoperative mobility and recovery are concerned.

Problems

However, there are two problems associated with obesity.

DIFFICULTIES INDUCING A PNEUMOPERITONEUM

These arise due to the thickness of the subcutaneous fat and particularly of the extraperitoneal fat. The peritoneum is only loosely attached to the fascia and tends to push away in front of the Verres needle and trocars. This is a particular problem if the needle track is oblique and if it is below the umbilical scar (Fig. 9.1).

Below the umbilicus, the bladder expands up in the extraperitoneal space leaving the peritoneum particularly loose. Extraperitoneal insufflation of CO_2 is therefore more common in obese patients.

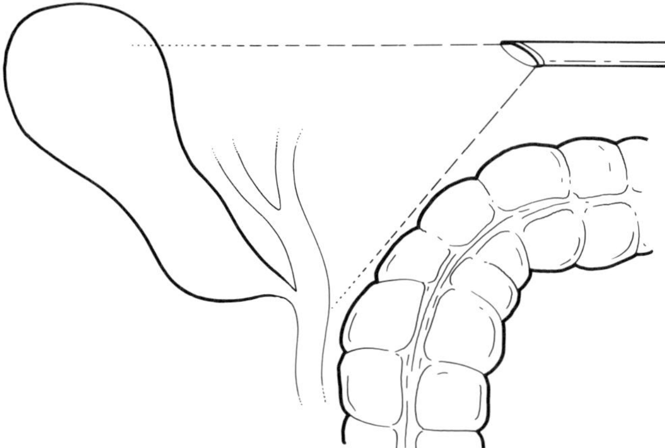

Fig. 9.2 The 30° scope can look over the top of the colon. This is especially helpful in obese patients.

Hints

1 We usually insufflate above the umbilicus where the peritoneum is more firmly fixed to the midline. This also has the advantage that the instruments are closer to the gallbladder. Lack of length of the Verres needle can be a problem in a very obese patient.

2 Pass the needle as near to a right angle to the skin surface as possible, lifting the skin and muscle together to angle it towards the pelvis.

OBESE COLON

Obese colon and omentum 'riding up' in front of the laparoscope during cholecystectomy and obscuring the view can be a problem.

Hints

1 The situation can be improved by lowering the patient's feet and rotating the patient to the left side so that the bulk of the viscera falls towards the left iliac fossa.

2 The most useful manoeuvre in our experience is to use the 30° laparoscope angled downwards so that it looks over the colon (Fig. 9.2).

3 Occasionally it is necessary to insert an extra port to retract the colon caudally.

4 Be sure to divide all adhesions to the under-surface of the liver as these hold the lower abdominal contents upwards obscuring the gallbladder bed (see p. 86).

Loss of pneumoperitoneum

The problem

The abdominal wall encroaches on the operative site due to a decrease in the pneumoperitoneum. Causes include the following.

1 Loss of relaxation; the effect of the relaxant drug has worn off.

2 Leak of CO_2 due to:

   (a) ports slipping out of abdominal wall,

   (b) open tap on a cannula,

   (c) prolonged aspiration with the sucker,

   (d) too large an incision around a port,

   (e) a torn rubber gasket on a port,

   (f) a reducing sleeve is holding the valve of a port open, or a reducing gasket has come loose from the cannula, or

   (g) instrument too small for the cannula or reducing device.

3 Failure of insufflation due to:

   (a) the port containing the air inlet has slipped out of the peritoneal cavity; this is easily overlooked,

   (b) the CO_2 line is blocked, or

   (c) the CO_2 cylinder is empty.

Hints

1 Check that CO_2 is emerging from the input line.

2 Check the tone of the abdominal muscles.

3 Listen for CO_2 leaks.

4 Check all cannula taps.

5 Review all rubber gaskets.

6 Check the position of the gas inlet cannula.

Haemorrhage

Bleeding from ports

The problem

Bleeding from the skin wounds around ports is common but not usually serious. It is worth cauterizing a cutaneous bleeder before inserting the cannula.

Bleeding from the deeper layers can be much more troublesome. This is often due to injury to the epigastric vessels running in the posterior part of the rectus sheath. Blood tends to trickle down the cannula and can splash over the laparoscope obscuring the view.

Such bleeding is commonly from one of the midline ports and is more likely if the port is slightly lateral to the midline.

Hints

1 Keep the trocar in the midline and only turn laterally to enter the peritoneal layer (see Fig. 7.17, p. 84).

2 Upwards and lateral pressure with a cannula can compress the artery. If this is maintained for 2 minutes it may cease to bleed.

3 Some surgeons pass a large curved needle through all layers of the abdomen, pick it up internally with a grasper or needle holder, and pass it out again on the other side of the bleeding point. This can then be tied externally over a gauze roll and removed near the end of the operation.

4 If the vessel continues to bleed, we prefer to enlarge the external incision slightly and under-run the bleeder under direct vision. The wound can then be closed round the cannula by deep sutures and the operation continued.

Retroperitoneal haematoma

The problem

On passing the laparoscope into the peritoneal cavity, a posterior wall haematoma is noted. There may or may not be fresh blood leaking into the peritoneal cavity. The haematoma is due to damage to a retroperitoneal vessel on the posterior abdominal wall. Similar haematomata may also be produced in the mesentery of the bowel. The injury is usually due to a trocar impinging on the posterior abdominal wall and is more common in thin patients.

Hints

1 In almost all cases, the abdomen will have to be opened and the bleeding controlled. Urgent action may be required. Patients have died due to hesitation by the surgeon. Call for the laparotomy set (which should always be available in theatre) and open the abdomen through a midline incision.

2 Having opened the abdomen, assess the point of haemorrhage. If it looks possible that there is a caval injury, there will be a danger of air embolism when the vessel is exposed. Tilt the patient head down and ask the anaesthetist to keep the venous pressure positive. Expose

the bleeding point if necessary by slitting the posterior peritoneum until the vessel is seen. Apply pressure with a pack and maintain it. The situation is now under control and blood can be replaced.

3 Send for the surgeon who is most competent to repair major vascular injuries. Attempts to repair the vena cava by inexperienced surgeons can result in fatal haemorrhage. The vessel must be carefully controlled above and below the site of the leak and the laceration sutured with fine vascular sutures. More minor vessel injuries are easier to deal with.

4 Adequate suction is essential. Two suckers are usually required.

Major haemorrhage into the peritoneal cavity, origin unclear

The problem

There is a steadily increasing pool of blood in the peritoneum, the origin of which is not clear.

Hints

Warn the anaesthetist blood may be required. Call for the laparotomy set. If the situation is stable:

1 Check the retroperitoneum. There may be a haematoma hidden behind loops of small bowel. If so proceed as above.

2 Check the cannula entry sites. One of them may be bleeding (see p. 112).

3 Check any adhesions which have been divided. A bleeding vessel can slip away from the operation site unnoticed. Control it with a preformed catgut ligature, clip or diathermy as seems appropriate.

4 Review the porta hepatis. A clip may have slipped off the cystic artery.

Major haemorrhage from hepatic or cystic arteries, or portal vein

The problem

A major vessel is perforated during dissection. Blood may spray over the end of the laparoscope obscuring the view. The posterior abdominal cavity fills up with blood and irrigation fluid, covering the vital structures. Because of the magnification involved, such bleeders look terrifying but they do not necessarily mean instant conversion to open surgery.

Hints

1 This problem is best avoided by taking more care over the dissection, and seeking and controlling vessels before they are cut. Being careful may take longer but if a major bleed is encountered a lot more time will be lost.

2 Make sure a laparotomy set and vascular instruments are available in theatre. If the patient's blood pressure falls or you are not controlling the situation, convert to open surgery. Then apply pressure and control the bleeding in the conventional way.

3 It is often possible to control the situation laparoscopically. Apply pressure by replacing the tissue or organ you were dissecting at the time of encountering the vessel. For instance, you may press the gallbladder back into the liver bed over the top of the bleeder. Remove and clean the laparoscope to restore the view. Replace it and review the situation from a distance. If the bleeding is not controlled you may be able to see where to reapply the pressure. Once the situation is controlled by pressure, insert the suction irrigator, wash in saline and then suck out the clot. Be sure you have enough irrigating fluid. Maintain pressure on the bleeder throughout.

Once the area is clean, release the pressure gradually and note the precise site of the bleeding. Reapply the pressure before too much blood escapes. It may be necessary to repeat this several times until the bleeding site is defined. Make a mental note of the angle and depth at which a haemostatic clip should be applied. Remove the sucker and place the clip accordingly. This can often be done even when the view is obscured by blood. A multiple clip applier is useful.

In summary. Keep cool, apply pressure, clean the area, get control. If you are losing, open the patient.

Haemorrhage from the gallbladder bed

The problem
There is persistent bleeding from the gallbladder bed after the gallbladder has been freed.

Hints
1 Use a button diathermy probe as on p. 16.
2 Use a laser to produce rosettes of deeper burns around the vessel (see Fig. 4.12, p. 46).

3 A roll of a haemostatic material (such as Surgicel, Gelfoam or Novacol) can be passed into the peritoneum and held against the bleeding point until coagulation occurs.
4 Use the detached gallbladder to provide pressure.
5 Fold the gallbladder bed over using closed graspers pressed on the liver surface. This form of pressure narrows the open sinusoids and is often remarkably successful.

Problems due to inflammation and fibrosis

Peritoneal adhesions

Insufflation and cannulation in the presence of peritoneal adhesions
Peritoneal adhesions from previous surgery or peritonitis can produce major difficulties, both in insufflating and initial cannulation of the abdomen, and in displaying and removing the gallbladder.

The first problem is to enter the peritoneum without damaging a loop of adherent bowel.

Technique
An attempt may be made to insufflate normally (as on p. 37).

The initial incision and Verres needle insertion should be away from previous abdominal scars if possible. Go above the umbilicus if the previous scar is below. If the needle does not move freely inside the peritoneal cavity, or if there is a rapid rise in inflow pressure and a fall in flow, stop insufflating. Try inserting the needle in another direction, such as upwards to the left hypochondrium or right hypochondrium. If this is still unsatisfactory proceed as below.

CUT DOWN INSUFFLATION
Keeping the incision as small as possible, cut down through the skin and fat to visualize the linea alba. Use two small retractors and scissors to deepen the wound under direct vision. When the linea alba is visible, make a small craniocaudal incision in it. The extraperitoneal fat appears. Part it by blunt dissection until the peritoneum is seen. At this stage, introduce a cannula with a blunt-ended trocar or without a trocar. Remove the trocar and pass the laparoscope down the cannula and inspect the peritoneum. It is usually possible to see an area of translucent peritoneum with free lying

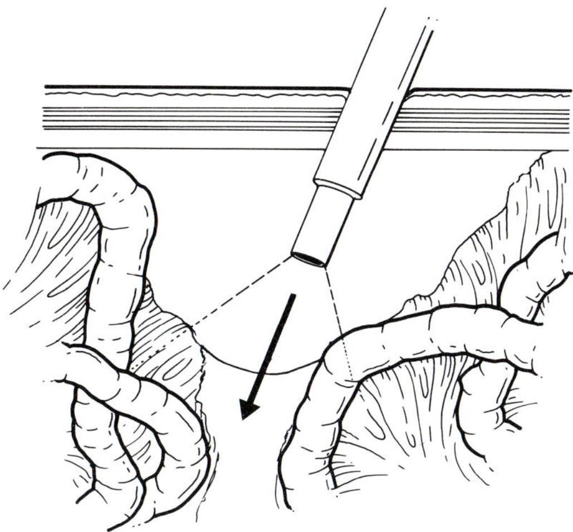

Fig. 9.3 When caught in a pocket of peritoneum isolated by adhesions, the laparoscope can be used to find a way into the main peritoneal cavity.

bowel (mobile) beyond it. Penetrate the peritoneum at this point and insufflate through the cannula.

If the hole made is now too big for the cannula, allowing escape of gas, place full thickness sutures on both sides of the wound and then re-insert the cannula between them. When the sutures are tied, the leak should be controlled. An alternative is to use the Hasson cork cannula (see p. 5).

Once insufflation has been achieved introduce a second cannula under direct vision. Instruments in this second port can then be used to divide further adhesions until the peritoneum can be inspected and the gallbladder exposed.

Dangers

1 In the initial stages, it is easy to penetrate a loop of bowel stuck to the peritoneum under the wound. If this is done, the wound should be enlarged and the hole sutured. If the bowel laceration is extensive, an open laparotomy may be essential.

2 You may enter an isolated pocket of peritoneum. In that case, advance the laparoscope and make a new hole between adhesions to enter the wider peritoneal cavity (Fig. 9.3).

3 It is also possible to mistake the extraperitoneal space for adhesions within the peritoneal cavity. In the extraperitoneal space,

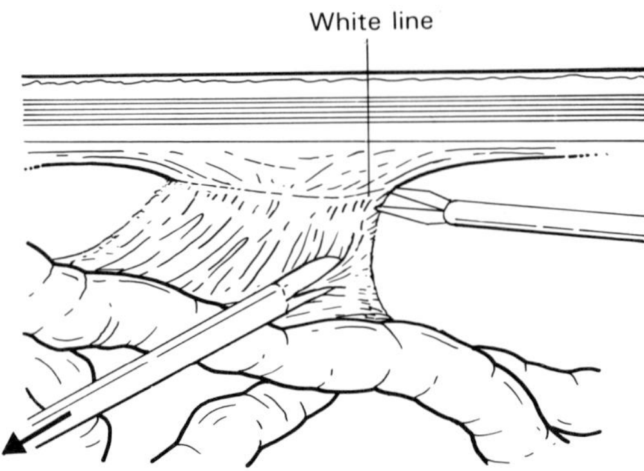

Fig. 9.4 The method of dividing peritoneal adhesions: put the adhesion on the stretch and divide the white line at the point of attachment to the parietal peritoneum or to the bowel.

however, there is a fine filamentous cobweb of strands as opposed to the sheets of adhesions in an adherent peritoneum.

Hints
Be patient, careful and persistent and you will find a workable peritoneal cavity.

Other problems due to adhesions
Apart from difficulties in initiating laparoscopy, adhesions within the abdomen may:
   (a) obscure the view of the gallbladder,
   (b) prevent full distension and retraction of the abdominal wall,
   (c) prevent access to the cystic duct and porta hepatis.

Hints
1 Put the adhesions on the stretch and divide them using scissors and/or diathermy (or laser) close to the parietal peritoneum or to the organ of origin. Most adhesions are avascular, and under tension a thin white line can be seen where they tent up the peritoneum at the point of attachment. Divide along this line (Fig. 9.4).
2 Keep hold of the adhesion until you are sure that the divided edge is not bleeding.
3 Light adhesions to the gallbladder can often be 'stripped down' by blunt dissection. In separating adhesions between the colon or duodenum, and gallbladder, grasp the bowel gently and put the

adhesions on the stretch. Cut very close to the gallbladder wall and gradually extract it from the adherent structures.

Adherent duodenum and colon

The problem
The colon and duodenum are firmly stuck to the anterior and inferior surface of the gallbladder, obscuring the view of Calot's triangle. There is a danger that they, or the gallbladder, will be perforated as the two structures are freed. Occasionally there may even be a pre-existing fistula.

Hints
1 Grasp the colon or duodenum with atraumatic graspers and try to define the layer between the bowel and the gallbladder. If necessary reapply the graspers several times until you can see an area to divide.
2 Use sharp dissection (scissors) and keep close to the gallbladder wall. It is better to open the gallbladder than the bowel.
3 Sometimes an 'outflanking manoeuvre' is possible. Approach the problem area from a new direction, from above or below the gallbladder for instance, and develop a plane from that area.
4 The management of a hole in the gallbladder is discussed on p. 123.
5 The management of a hole in the bowel is discussed on p. 121.

Small shrunken gallbladder

The problem
This is probably one of the most difficult problems to deal with particularly if the organ is deep in the liver. It may be difficult to grasp the gallbladder wall, and difficult to retract the gallbladder to achieve dissection between it and the liver. This kind of pathology may necessitate abandoning the laparoscopic operation and converting to open surgery. The gallbladder remains difficult and hazardous to remove even under direct vision.

Hints
1 If necessary, replace one of the 5 mm ports with a 10 mm port and

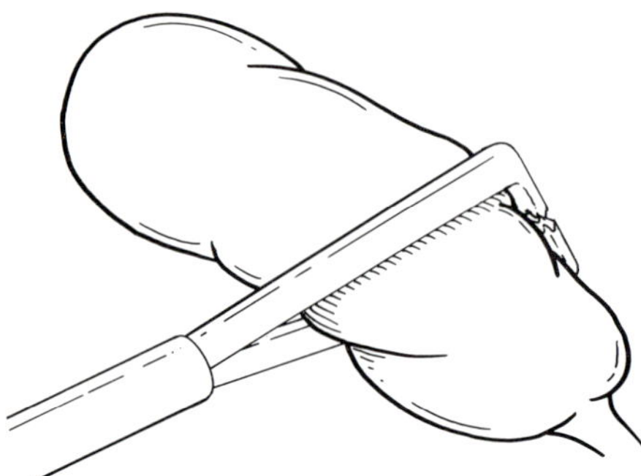

Fig. 9.5 Using a 10 mm crocodile jaw graspers on a non-compressible gallbladder.

insert large traumatic claw graspers (see p. 20) to grip the gall-bladder. They may make a hole in the wall but this is preferable to abandoning the operation (Fig. 9.5).

2 See also below under Empyema of the gallbladder, Fibrosis around the portal triad and Oedematous thickened gallbladder wall.

Empyema of the gallbladder

The problem
This gives rise to similar difficulties with the additional hazards of increased oozing and a tense gallbladder full of pus.

Hints
1 Extensive use of the diathermy and irrigation are necessary to expose the gallbladder. Dilated small vessels bleed persistently.
2 It may be advantageous to empty the gallbladder deliberately (as on p. 125) before doing so accidentally during dissection.

Fibrosis around the portal triad

The problem
There is such extensive fibrosis around the cystic duct that it is impossible to define this structure without the risk of damaging the common bile duct or the cystic duct itself. This can occur where there is a stone stuck in the cystic duct or Hartmann's pouch, with associated severe inflammation.

Hints
1 It can be helpful to develop a layer more laterally behind

Hartmann's pouch (in safety) and then extend it medially to define the cystic duct. Keep very close to the gallbladder wall, dividing all vessels as they enter the wall and do not worry about the main trunks.

2 In extreme cases, it may be necessary to divide the gallbladder at this level and suture around the cystic duct opening while viewing it from inside the gallbladder. The distal gallbladder can then be excised if necessary leaving the posterior wall attached to the liver. A contact laser is very useful in this kind of surgery.

3 The fragments of the gallbladder, and any stones, can be collected up into a bag (see pp. 96–7) and removed.

Oedematous thickened gallbladder wall

The problem
The gallbladder wall is so thickened, oedematous and rigid that graspers keep slipping off it.

Hints
1 The situation may be helped by emptying the gallbladder as on p. 125.
2 If all else fails, do not hesitate to exchange the subcostal 5 mm port for a 10 mm port and insert a pair of 10 mm claw tooth graspers (see p. 20). These can be used to encircle the gallbladder or allow a grip on its wall even at the expense of perforation. Such thickened gallbladders often do not spill stones very easily and even if they do, retrieving them is a better option than converting to open surgery.

Problems due to surgical trauma

Verres needle or trocar injuries
These include perforation of the bowel (see below), penetration of the retroperitoneal structures (see Retroperitoneal haematoma, p. 113), and intraperitoneal haemorrhage (p. 114). These are dealt with in the relevant sections.

Damage to the bowel

The problem
Either the small or large bowel can be damaged by the Verres needle, a trocar, or in freeing adhesions to gain access to the gallbladder.

Hints

1 The most important step is to recognize that the injury has occurred. Suspect a hole in the bowel if the fluid in the peritoneal cavity looks unusually murky or green or brown. Usually the hole will be recognized as soon as it is made.

2 A small fresh hole in the bowel can be sutured laparoscopically, providing the surgeon has the necessary expertise and provided the edges are fresh and clean (see p. 52).

3 In any other circumstances the abdomen should be opened and the bowel repaired and the cholecystectomy completed under direct vision.

Damage to hepatic or common bile ducts

The problem

The main biliary tract can be damaged in a number of ways, particularly if there is confusion about the real anatomy (see Chapter 7, pp. 69–74). The injury will be apparent when bile is seen to be leaking from an unexpected site.

Hints

1 The injury should be carefully visualized. If there is a clean straight cut in the common bile duct, a T-tube can be inserted and the laceration closed over it (as on p. 105).

2 If the precise nature of the injury is not clear or the tear is ragged or extensive, the abdomen should be opened and a repair carried out under direct vision. This should be done by the most senior hepato-biliary surgeon available. If the duct mucosa is largely intact, a T-tube is inserted as above. If the segment of duct is irretrievably damaged or missing it may be necessary to insert a loop of jejunum. Where there is doubt, a T-tube is the preferred option with a later secondary repair when the duct system will be more dilated.

3 If the cystic artery has not been divided, a vascularized patch of gallbladder can be fashioned as a conduit or a patch to repair damage to the common bile duct wall.

Postoperative care

After a bile duct injury, a T-tube should be left in place for at least a month and removed after a T-tube cholangiogram confirms that the duct system is patent. The patient should then be followed up regularly for several years. If symptoms of biliary obstruction or cholangitis develop, an endoscopic retrograde cholangiogram should be performed. Late stricture should be referred to an expert hepato-biliary surgeon and repaired under optimum circumstances.

Hole in the gallbladder

The problem
The gallbladder wall is perforated during dissection allowing escape of bile and/or stones. A perforated gallbladder may spill further stones during extraction.

Hints
1 A very small hole leaking bile only may be of little consequence though the peritoneum should be carefully washed out afterwards.
2 A slightly larger hole can be closed with a clip or clips. Pick up and appose the edges with graspers and then apply a clip to hold them together.
3 Two clips can be applied to the hole at right angles to each other.
4 An alternative is to insert the sucker in the gallbladder and aspirate most of the bile. Insert a catgut loop ligature, pass a grasper through it and pick up the edges of the perforation. The loop can then be tightened, thus sealing the perforation.

The problem of spilling stones during extraction of the gallbladder is dealt with below.

Loss of stones in the peritoneum

The problem
The gallbladder is perforated and one or several stones spill into the peritoneal cavity. Large stones may be too big to extract through even a 10 mm port.

Hints
1 Although it is obviously tidier to remove such stones, most surgeons have had this experience and to date complications due to leaving stones in the peritoneal cavity have not been reported.
2 If a large number of stones are lost, it can be useful to insert a bag

(see p. 96) and collect up the loose stones into this. This is more efficient than removing each stone separately. The bag can be left in the abdomen until the end of the operation and the gallbladder also placed in it prior to extraction.

3 Small stones can be removed with a sucker and larger bore suckers have been designed especially for this purpose. The stones do, however, tend to get stuck in the valve of the suction probe or block the tubing.

4 Stone extracting forceps are available with a 10 mm shaft and large cupped jaws (Chapter 2, p. 20).

CO_2 embolism

The problem

This can occur if a large hepatic sinusoid is opened in the gallbladder bed. The CO_2 in the peritoneum is under positive pressure and may enter the venous system. CO_2 can also be injected into veins under pressure when using a contact tip laser cooled with a jet of CO_2. If the tip is pressed into hepatic tissue, the CO_2 exit port can enter a vein. The diagnosis is picked up by the anaesthetist noticing a change in the end-tidal CO_2 levels and deterioration in patient condition.

Hints

The problem is deal with on p. 64.

Loss of a needle in the peritoneal cavity

The problem

After suturing, a needle is dropped before or during extraction from one of the laparoscopic ports and is not immediately apparent.

Hints

1 Do nothing immediately. The needle is probably lying on a loop of bowel somewhere and will remain there unless the peritoneal contents are disturbed. Check that it is not caught on one of the cannulae. If you are using a 30° laparoscope, it may be useful to change to a 0° laparoscope for initial inspection of the peritoneal cavity. Move the laparoscope to another port if this will help.

2 Inspect the area directly beneath the relevant port. The needle

may be seen glinting in the transmitted light. If careful inspection in all areas fails to reveal it, pass a grasper through another port and very gently move the loops of bowel under the relevant port aside, disturbing the peritoneal contents as little as possible with each manoeuvre. Progress slowly and carefully and the needle will usually be found.

3 If it still remains hidden, place two graspers through separate ports and align them on some point on the posterior abdominal wall, take an abdominal X-ray and note the relative position of the needle and the graspers.

4 An alternative is to place three metal clips as markers.

Once the needle has been found, grasp the loose end of suture and extract it through the port. Do not attempt to extract it holding the needle itself as this will often impact against the edge of the port causing you to drop it. If it is held by the thread, the needle is free to follow the path of least resistance.

Anatomical and pathological difficulties

Distended gallbladder

The problem
The gallbladder is so tense and distended that graspers slip off it and traction seems impossible.

Hints
1 It is often possible to find a fold of mesentery close to the liver and apply graspers to that rather than the gallbladder itself.
2 Repeated attempts at grasping, passing from one instrument to another, may empty some bile and allow a fold of wall to be gripped.
3 The gallbladder may be emptied using a needle or a 5 mm port stuck into the fundus. The midclavicular port is suitable. The hole created can then be gripped with the fundal graspers, or tied off with a preformed catgut ligature, to minimize further leakage.

Intrahepatic gallbladder

The problem
The gallbladder is situated deep in the liver and almost surrounded

by hepatic tissue. This makes it difficult to free from the liver, the plane of dissection appearing to be at the 'wrong angle' to the operative port. Sometimes only an area of the fundus is intrahepatic and may protrude onto the superior surface of the liver.

Hints

1 Divide the peritoneum between the gallbladder and the liver along both edges of the gallbladder. Having divided the cystic duct and artery, apply traction close to the liver attachments and divide the strands as they become visible. Proceeding in this way the gallbladder can gradually be enucleated from the enclosing liver tissue.
2 Always keep close to the gallbladder wall. There is a danger of opening hepatic sinusoids by dissecting too deep into the liver.
3 If the dissection becomes too difficult on one side, move to the opposite side of the gallbladder. Keep moving from place to place cutting strands where the edge of the gallbladder is better defined.

Abnormal anatomy
This subject is dealt with on pp. 69–74.

Stones in the cystic duct

The problem
Stones in the cystic duct may make it impossible to pass a cholangiogram catheter more than a few millimetres. They may also be pushed into the common bile duct during dissection and clipping of the cystic duct.

Hints

1 Suspect stones in the cystic duct if it looks wide or non-compressible.
2 Place clips on the distal end of the duct to prevent further stones coming down from the gallbladder. Open the duct and apply atraumatic graspers medially and milk the duct contents towards the opening.
3 A temporary clip placed medially can prevent stones slipping into the common duct during manipulation of the cystic duct.
4 Sometimes it is necessary to extend the cystic duct opening down towards the stone with microscissors.
5 If one stone is removed check whether there are any more. They are often multiple.

6 When the duct is clear, clean bile can be seen flowing from the opening.

Stones in the common bile duct
See Chapter 8, pp. 100–7.

Short cystic duct

The problem
The cystic duct is very short leading to problems in defining, cannulating, and closing it.

Hints
1 Some of the difficulties defining a short cystic duct are discussed in Chapter 7 (pp. 69–71).
2 Dissect as far up the gallbladder as possible and cannulate Hartmann's pouch if necessary.
3 It may be impossible to apply two clips safely to the duct medially though this is unusual. In that case, hold the gallbladder neck with graspers, divide the duct as far laterally as possible including part of the gallbladder neck, and close the duct with a preformed catgut ligature. It may also be necessary to ligate the neck of the gallbladder in the same way.
4 If a short cystic duct breaks off close to the hepatic ducts, it may be necessary to close it with a suture through its origin.

Wide cystic duct

The problem
The cystic duct is too wide to close with metal clips.

Hints
1 There may be stones in the cystic duct medially. Check as above and do an operative cholangiogram.
2 There may be stones in the common bile duct (see Chapter 8).
3 Either (a) pass a ligature around the duct, tie an internal (p. 54) or external (p. 49) knot, and close the duct; or (b) divide the duct, holding the medial end with graspers. Pass a previously prepared

catgut loop ligature down a port and regrasp the duct through the loop. Snug the knot down and cut off the excess (see p. 51).

Large stones

The problem

A gallstone larger than 1 cm cannot be extracted through the abdominal wounds.

Hints

1 The stone can sometimes be crushed within the gallbladder once it has been brought to the surface. Heavy straight artery forceps, or a specially designed lithotripter forceps may be used for this. The fragments of the stone can then be extracted.

2 If available, an ultrasonic or electrostatic shock wave lithotripters can be used to break up large stones. The probe is held against the stone, activated, and the stone shattered.

3 We will not hesitate to enlarge the skin and muscle layer incision in order to extract a large stone if it cannot easily be broken up. This is described in Chapter 7, p. 97.

Difficult extraction

The problem

Extraction may be difficult due to subcutaneous obesity, large gallstones, or due to the likelihood of rupture of a thin-walled or damaged gallbladder. In the latter case, stones may drop out of the gallbladder as it is pulled through the abdominal incision.

Medium-sized (10–15 mm) stones may impact in the extraction port because they line up side by side at right angles to the port.

Hints

1 The danger from loss of stones is lessened if the gallbladder is extracted through the epigastric port. Any stones that fall then lie on the liver and can be more easily retrieved. Stones falling beneath the umbilical port fall in loops of bowel and may be difficult to find.

2 Use of a bag to extract the gallbladder. It can be very useful to insert a bag into the abdomen, place the gallbladder within it, and extract the bag containing the gallbladder. This has the advantage

that any stones falling out of the gallbladder during the compression experienced during extraction, fall within the bag and not within the peritoneal cavity. Various bags have been used by different surgeons. We initially used a thin-walled plastic bag. This could tear under extreme traction. Other surgeons have used a sterilized condom. H. Espiner of Bristol has designed a special bag made out of hot air balloon fabric. This can be autoclaved. Its use is described in Chapter 7, p. 96.

3 Medium-sized stones can often be realigned using a closed grasper to manipulate the gallbladder from inside the abdomen. Once in line, they can be extracted without enlarging the port. Loosen the traction on the gallbladder while this is achieved.

Collapse of patient

The problem
The patient may collapse due to the following.
1 Haemorrhage. This may be already apparent or may be unsuspected and retroperitoneal. The problem is dealt with on pp. 112–14.
2 CO_2 embolus (pp. 64, 124).
3 Excessive intraperitoneal gas pressure causing loss of venous return. Check the insufflation pressure and open one of the ports.
4 Drug reaction. These are in the province of the anaesthetist and will not be dealt with here.

Hints
If a collapse occurs:
1 Discontinue insufflation and ensure by palpation of the abdomen that the peritoneal pressure is not too high.
2 Decide quickly whether unsuspected bleeding could be a cause. Inspect the retroperitoneum. Inspect the whole peritoneal cavity.
3 Proceed according to the cause of the collapse as indicated on the pages above.

10: Postoperative course

Pain

Analgesia

Oro-gastric tube

Urinary catheter

Drains

Oral fluids

Oral feeding

Mobility and convalescence

Follow-up

Introduction

The most important difference between open cholecystectomy and laparoscopic cholecystectomy is the ease of the postoperative course. A proportion of patients (20% in our series) are able to leave on the same day as the surgery and most of the rest leave on the morning after the operation. It is useful to keep the first few patients of a series in longer than this so that the surgeon and staff can gain confidence in the rapidity of recovery and be able to advise future patients as to what to expect.

Patients do vary widely in their speed of recovery and symptoms after operation and it is difficult to predict an individual patient's course. It does not seem to be related to the length of anaesthetic or the difficulty of the operative procedure. Indeed, some of our patients who have complained of the most pain postoperatively have had the easiest and quickest operations.

Pain

1 Most patients mention some right upper quadrant discomfort which is usually described as moderate but very occasionally as severe. In the majority of cases the pain is relieved by mild analgesics such as paracetamol or diclofenac.

2 Shoulder tip pain is felt by about half the patients. It is rarely severe. It also occurs after laparoscopies for gynaecological procedures and must therefore be related to the pneumoperitoneum rather than the gallbladder operation. It settles over 2 or 3 days. The patients should be warned about it and reassured that it is not serious. We have formed the impression that draining off the carbon dioxide and residual peritoneal fluid in the few hours after the operation results in less shoulder tip pain.

3 Pain in one or other of the stab wounds is not uncommon. It settles very rapidly. Increasing pain after 2 or 3 days may be a sign of infection and occasionally antibiotics are indicated.

4 Persistent pain and increased requirement for opiates usually indicates a postoperative problem and these patients should be kept

under observation until the pain settles or its cause becomes apparent and treatment is instituted. Possible causes of prolonged pain include subhepatic haematoma formation, subhepatic biliary collection and residual stones in the common bile duct.

Analgesia

All our patients are given a diclofenac suppository with the premedication. In some patients this seems to be sufficient and no further analgesia is required. The majority do, however, require between one and four doses of 1 g paracetamol postoperatively. A smaller percentage of patients require opioid analgesia, either one or two doses postoperatively.

Oro-gastric tube

An oro-gastric tube is placed during the operation in order to keep the stomach empty. It should be removed as soon as the operation is over and before the patient wakes up.

Urinary catheter

If a catheter has been left in during the operation, it should be removed before the patient wakes up. Urinary retention is much less of a problem after laparoscopic surgery than after open laparotomy.

Drains

It is our practice to drain the peritoneum routinely. As mentioned above, we believe this decreases postoperative shoulder pain. Nevertheless, the drain itself can cause pain and we like to remove it as soon as drainage ceases, often within 1 or 2 hours of completing the operation.

If there has been suspected or actual damage to the biliary tree or excessive bleeding from the gallbladder bed, we will leave it longer and remove it sometime after 12 hours depending on the drainage.

The drain is a useful method of detecting continued postoperative haemorrhage. Continued blood loss in the first 1 or 2 hours postoperatively is an indication to return to theatre for an open laparotomy.

Oral fluids

There is no significant ileus after laparoscopic cholecystectomy and patients can start taking oral fluids as soon as they are awake. They usually do so 4–6 hours after the end of the operation.

Oral feeding

Providing the patient has a desire for it, a light meal can be taken 6 hours after the operation. Some patients remain slightly nauseated at this stage but almost all eat a normal breakfast on the morning after the operation.

Mobility and convalescence

Patients can get out of bed to go to the toilet as soon as they have recovered from the anaesthetic and they should be encouraged to do so. Such movements are remarkably pain-free when compared with the mobility achieved after an open operation. Similarly, patients can cough actively and clear bronchial secretions and hence there is a lower incidence of chest infection. As already indicated, many patients are able to walk out of hospital on the evening of their operation and almost all are fully mobile by the following morning. Thereafter, the postoperative recovery is variable. Some patients prefer to take things quietly for the first 2 or 3 days, interspersing increasing exercise with rests. After the third day, patients have undertaken increasing amounts of activity. Some have played golf or gone to yoga classes by the fifth postoperative day. Others have taken rather longer to resume a normal lifestyle. The average return to work in our series is 9.2 days. This includes a few patients who have opted to take an extra 1 or 2 weeks off work for their own reasons.

Follow-up

Because the patient is discharged so quickly, we find it helpful to see them in outpatients within a week or 10 days of surgery. In most cases this appointment is an occasion for mutual congratulation but a significant number of important queries can also be dealt with. Some patients (and their relatives) require added reassurance that it is safe to undertake normal activity.

We review the patients finally after another 6 weeks but ask them to return if they develop further upper abdominal pain or jaundice. In that case an upper abdominal ultrasound (to look for collections or for bile duct obstruction) is carried out, together with liver function tests. So far, we have not found any significant problems at late follow-up, but the known incidence of hepatic duct damage (about 0.3% in open surgery, possibly 0.6% in laparoscopic surgery) means clinicians should always look out for such problems.

Appendix: Handout for patients

CHOLECYSTECTOMY
Your gallbladder operation — some information

What is a gallbladder? The gallbladder lies behind your right ribs at the front, under the liver and above the duodenum (gut). It is a pouch connected with the tubing (bile duct) which carries bile from the liver to the gut. It acts as a reservoir for bile. Stones forming in the gallbladder often cause pain. If stones escape from the gallbladder they can block the bile duct and cause pain, fever and yellow jaundice. They may also cause inflammation in the pancreatic gland — a condition called pancreatitis.

Treatment of gallstones. Attempts can be made to remove gallstones from the gallbladder by medical treatment or by shattering them by lithotripsy. Many stones do not respond to medical treatment however. Even those that do may take up to 2 years of treatment and this treatment itself causes symptoms in the form of colicky abdominal pain and diarrhoea. Lithotripsy shatters the gallstones and this causes them to leave the gallbladder and may then cause complications associated with blockage of the bile duct (see above). A big disadvantage of treatments involving removal of stones rather than removing the gallbladder itself, is that stones reform. Damage to the gallbladder wall by the stones results in further crystallization after the stones are removed. The best treatment for gallstones is therefore to remove the damaged gallbladder together with the stones. The operation is called cholecystectomy.

Conventional cholecystectomy. In a conventional cholecystectomy the abdomen is opened through a cut in the skin below the right ribs at the front. The gallbladder and its stones are removed and X-rays are taken to show whether there are any stones in the bile duct. If there are they are removed. The cut in the skin is then closed up.

Laparoscopic cholecystectomy. In a laparoscopic cholecystectomy only tiny stab wounds 5–10 mm in length are made in the abdomen. There may be four or occasionally five of these. Through one of these (usually next to the navel) a telescope (laparoscope) is inserted and a video camera attached to it. This projects a picture of the internal organs onto a television screen. Instruments are then passed through the other small stab wounds and using the picture on the screen the surgeon is able to free the gallbladder from its attachments to the liver without actually opening the abdomen further.

During the operation the surgeon may carry out an X-ray to visualize the bile ducts and see whether there are any stones in them. It may also be possible to remove these, but if this is not possible there are two options. The first is to abandon the laparoscopic approach, make a normal incision and remove the stone. The surgeon will avoid doing this unless the stones are very large. The second is to leave the stones where they are and arrange a special procedure to be done after the operation (endoscopy). This involves passing a flexible telescope down through the stomach into the first part of the bowel, inspecting the lower end of the bile duct and removing any stones that may be in it. This does not require an abdominal incision. Many stones can be removed from the bile duct in this way. If there is a stone which it is impossible to remove this way then again there may be a need for a later operation. This is very rare, however.

Postoperative recovery. After a conventional cholecystectomy the patient usually stays in hospital between 7 and 10 days and returns to work after 6 weeks. After a laparoscopic cholecystectomy the patient is usually ready to go home within 24 hours and can return to full activity including work within 10–14 days, occasionally even sooner.

Before the operation. Take light meals on the day before your admission. You should have nothing to eat or drink at all for 6 hours before the operation is due to start. You will be asked to hand in any medicines or drugs you may be taking, so that your drug treatment in hospital will be correct. Please tell the nurses of any allergies to drugs or dressings.

Periods. Periods do not affect the operation.

Shaving. It will be helpful if you can shave all the hairs off your abdomen before you come into hospital.

Bowels. You will be given a suppository to insert in the anus before the operation. This is to empty the large bowel which can otherwise obstruct the surgeon's view.

The operation is then performed.

What happens after the operation? After a laparoscopic cholecystectomy a drainage tube may be left in the abdomen to empty off any residual gas or fluid from the abdominal cavity. This will usually be removed after 2–12 hours. Any skin clips or stitches will be removed on the day following the operation. You will also have an intravenous fluid drip in the arm when you return from theatre. This will be removed at about the same time as the drain.

Will if affect me to lose my gallbladder? There is no evidence that losing the gallbladder causes any side effects or symptoms. In fact you will be much better off without a diseased gallbladder containing stones. The storage function of the gallbladder is taken over by the remaining bile ducts after the operation.

Will it hurt? The wounds are slightly painful but not usually markedly so. You will be given painkillers if you need them. Ask for more if the pain is still unpleasant. Strong painkillers can increase the nausea you may feel after the operation. You will be expected to get out of bed the evening of the operation. You will not do the wounds any harm, and the exercise is very helpful for you. A proportion of patients have pain in the shoulder after a laparoscopy. This is not serious and settles over a few days.

Drinking and eating. You should be eating normally on the day after the operation. If you have not opened your bowels after 2 days and you feel uncomfortable, ask your doctor for a laxative.

The wounds. There may be some purple bruising around the wounds which spreads downwards by gravity and fades to a yellow colour after 2–3 days. It is not important. Occasionally minor matchhead-sized blebs form on the wound line, but these settle down after discharging a blob of yellow fluid for a day or so.

Washing. You can wash the wound areas gently after 48 hours. A little soap and tap water are entirely adequate. Salted water is not necessary. Keep the wounds dry at other times.

Sick notes. Please ask your GP for sick notes, certificates, etc.

After you leave hospital. You are likely to feel slightly tired but this will improve over 3–5 days.

Driving. You can drive as soon as you can make an emergency stop without discomfort in the wound, i.e. after about 2 days.

What about sex? You can restart sexual relations after a few days when the wounds are comfortable enough.

Work. You should be able to return to a light job after about 5 days, and any heavy job within 2 weeks.

Complications. Complications are unusual.

If you think that all is not well, please ask your GP who will contact the hospital if necessary. Wound infection is a rare problem and settles down with antibiotics in a few days. Aches and twinges may be felt in the wound for a few weeks.

Index

Page numbers in *italics* refer to figures

abdominal organs, initial
  inspection 40–1
abdominal scars 56–7
abdominal surgery, previous, as
  contraindication 56–7
abdominal wall, retraction 41
Absolok 24, 25
adhesions
  colon 119
  as contraindication 57
  dividing 86–7, 118
  duodenal 119
  gallbladder 86–7
  peritoneal 116–19
advice sheet 60, 134–5
air, in insufflation 10
air embolism 64
alkaline phosphatase, raised levels 58,
  100
anaesthesia
  operative management 62–5
  postoperative management 65–7
  pre-operative management 59,
    61–2
anaesthestist, position 74
analgesics
  postoperative 66, 130, 131
  pre-operative 59, 131
  systemic 66
anatomy
  normal 68–9
  variations 69–74
antibiotics, prophylactic 59, 65
anti-emetics, postoperative 65, 66
antithrombosis stockings 59, 74
aorta, penetration 40
argon lasers 32
atracurium 63
atraumatic forceps 20
atropine, prophylactic use 62

bags
  in gallbaldder extraction 96–7,
    128–9
  in retrieval of lost stones 123–4
balloon catheter, in removal of
    common duct stones 102–4
bare fibre lasers
  dangers 45
  technique 45, 46
baskets 26–7, 104–5
benzodiazepines, pre-operative 61

Betadine 78
biliary tract
  damage to 27, 122–3
  stones 100–7
bilirubin, raised levels 58, 100
bisacodyl 58
bladder
  catheterization 59, 65, 77, 131
  pre-operative emptying 59, 65
blindness, laser-induced 31
blood, loss assessment 64
blood warmer, as laparoscope
    warmer 13–14
blunt dissection, techniques 46–7
bowel, damage to 80–1, 121–2
bradycardia 62
bupivicaine 65
burning, inadvertent 16

Calot's triangle
  dangers of diathermy in 43–4
  dissection around 22
  exposure 85
  obscured view of 6
camera 9
  image orientation 35, 36
  position 76
  sterilization 9, 79
camera–laparoscope interface,
    ventilation 9, 110
cannulae 1–2, 3
  Hasson cork 5, 117
cannulation
  extraperitoneal 81
  in presence of peritoneal
    adhesions 116–18
  subcutaneous 81
carbon dioxide (CO_2)
  absorption, monitoring 10
  embolism 40, 64, 124, 129
  in insufflation 10
  leakage 112
  surgical emphysema due to 40
  use in pressurizing irrigating
    fluid 23
carbon dioxide lasers 31–2
catgut 50
  preformed ligatures 50–1
catheter, cholangiography 26
cefotaxime 59, 65
chest infections 132
cholangiography

intravenous 58
operative 56, 58, 88–91, 101
cholangiography catheter 26
cholangiography clamp 26, 90
cholecystectomy
  open 100–1
    conversion to 60
cholecystitis, acute, history of 56
cholecystography, oral,
     pre-operative 57
choledocholithiasis, patient
    information 60
choledochotomy, common bile duct
    exploration through 105–6
choledoscopy, common bile duct
    exploration through 106–7
clamp, cholangiography 26, 90
clip applicators 24–5
  multiple 24–5, 48
clips 24
  Absolok 24, 25
  disposable 48–9
  incorrect placement 48
  in internal knot tying 55
  Ligaclip 24
  removal 48, 49
  self-locking 48–9
  techniques of use 47–9
coagulation *see* diathermy
colon
  adhesions 119
  obese 111
  pushing/pulling downwards 42
common bile duct
  anatomy 68
  damage to 72, 122–3
  dilation 57, 100, 103–4
  laparoscopic exploration 101–2
    through a choledochotomy 105–6
    under X-ray control 102–5
    using a flexible
      choledoscope 106–7
  mistaken for cystic duct 69, 70
  see also common duct stones
common duct stones 58, 100
  laparoscopic lithotripsy 107
  management 100–7
  residual 131
common hepatic duct, anatomy 68
conical trocar point 3
contact tip lasers 33–4
  dangers 46

hints 46
technique 45, 46
convalescence 132
conversion to open cholecystects 100
cook needle holder 20, 21
cut down insufflation 116–18
cystic arteries
  anatomy 69
  anterior 72, 73
  division 91–2
  haemorrhage from 114–15
  multiple short arteries 72–3
  occlusion 24
  separate anterior and posterior 73–4
cystic duct
  access obscured by adhesions 118
  anatomy 68
  defining 87–8
  encircling 70–1
  fibrosis around 120–1
  long 71–2
  occlusion 24
  opening 16
  oral cholecystography 57
  short 127
  small lumen 91
  stones in 126–7
  very short 69–70
  entering right hepatic duct 70–1
  wide 127–8
cystic lymph node 69

deep vein thrombosis, pre-operative
    prophylaxis 59
Desjardin's forceps 96
diaphragmatic irritation 66
diathermy
  current conduction through
    irrigating fluid 16
  instruments 15–16
  lead attachments 79
  machine position 76
  with scissors 44–5
  techniques 42–4
diathermy button probe 15–16
diathermy hook 15, 16
  dangers 43–4
  hints 44
  technique 42–3
diathermy plate, position 77
diathermy spade 15, 16
diclofenac 59, 61, 130, 131

dissecting instruments 21–2
dissection
    blunt, techniques 46–7
    techniques 42–6
Dormia basket 26–7, 104–5
double jaw mechanism, forceps 20
drains 131
    insertion 93–4
    removal 99
droperidol 66
drug reactions 129
Dulcolax 58
duodenum, adhesions 119

electrical connections 108
electrical interference 108
electrons, excitation 28
embolism, carbon dioxide 40, 64,
        124, 129
emphysema, surgical 40
empyema, gallbladder 120
endoscopic cholangiography 58, 101
endoscopic retrograde
        cholangiopancreatography 58,
        101
endoscopic sphincterotomy,
        precholecystectomy 100
epigastric vessels, damage to 112–13
ERCP 58, 101
Espiner bag 96–7, 123–4, 129
Ethibinder 50
examination 56–7
excitation pump 29
extraperitoneal space
    cannulation 81
    mistaken for adhesions 117–18
eyes, patients, taping 65

falciform lift 41–2
fallopian tube, grasping 19
fat, on lens 108–9
feeding, oral, postoperative 132
fibrosis, around portal triad 120–1
fixed retractors 79
flap valve, cannulae 1, 3
fluids, oral, postoperative intake 131
follow-up 132
forceps
    atraumatic 20
    Desjardin's 96
    holding/grasping 17–20, 21
    lithotripter 128

Petelin 21–2, 46
    stone extracting 20, 124
fore and aft technique 37
free movement test 39
'French position' 75

gallbladder
    adhesions 86–7
    anatomy 68
    distended 125
    emptying 125
        before retraction 85–6
    empyema 120
    extraction 95–6
        difficulties 128–9
        use of bag 96–7
    freeing from bed 92–3
    fundus 68
    haemorrhage from bed 115–16
    haemostasis of bed 93
    indications of functioning 57
    intrahepatic 57, 68, 125–6
    obscured by adhesions 118
    oedematous thickening 121
    perforation 123
    retraction 41, 85–6
    small shrunken 119–20
    on subhepatic mesentery 57
    tenderness over 57
    thin-walled 57
    wall thickening 57
gallbladder fundus, holding 18
    gastric distension,
        intra-operative 65
    Gelfoam 116
general anaesthesia 62
grasping forceps 17–20, 21

haematoma
    retroperitoneal 40, 113–14
    subhepatic 131
haemorrhage 59, 129
    cystic arteries 114–15
    from ports 112–13
    gallbladder bed 115–16
    hepatic arteries 114–15
    portal vein 114–15
    potential for 64
    of unclear origin 114
haemostasis 42–6, 93, 94
halide light source 8
hand instruments 15–27

handle mechanisms   17–18
handout   60, 134–5
hands, relative importance in
        laparoscopy   35–6
Hartmann's pouch
    anatomy   68
    holding   18
    stones in   57
Hasson cork cannula   5, 117
heat loss, intra-operative   62
heparin
    in irrigating fluid   23
    pre-operative prophylactic   59
hepatic arteries, haemorrhage
        from   114–15
hepatic artery, anatomy   69
hepatic bile duct
    damage to   122–3
    stones in   100–7
hepatic veins   92
history taking   56–7
holding forceps   17–20, 21
holding/grasping mechanisms   19–20,
    21
hook, look, cook technique   43
hooked scissors   16, 17
Hopkins rod–lens system   6
hypoxaemia   63

illumination   8
incision
    initial   38
    supraumbilical   38
indicators of operative ease   57
indicators of possible operative
        difficulty   56–7
inferior vena cava, penetration   40
informed consent   60
instruments, hand   15–27
insufflation
    cutdown   116–18
    equipment   10–13
    extraperitoneal   110
    failure of   112
    initial   39
    in presence of peritoneal
        adhesions   116–18
insufflator   10–13
    connections   78
    consequences of leaks   80
    position   76
    testing   79–80

intercostal nerves, block   65–6
intraperitoneal pressure
    high   13, 63, 129
    monitoring   10–11
intravenous cholangiography   58
investigations   57–8
irrigating fluid
    conduction of diathermy current
        through   16
    delivery   22–3
irrigation
    dangers   47
    technique   47
irrigation devices   22–3
    connections   78–9
    position   76

jaundice   56, 100
jaw types, grasping/holding
        forceps   19, 20, 21

knots
    external
        dangers   50
        hints   50
        technique   49–50
    internal, technique   53–5
KTP lasers   32
kyphosis   57

laparoscope–camera interface,
        ventilation   9, 110
laparoscopes
    defogging   109
    fogging   109–10
    forward viewing   6, 7
    operating   6–7
    side viewing   6, 7
    standard   6, 7
    warming   13–14, 109
    warming device   13–14
        position   76
laparoscopic techniques   37–55
    converting to   35–7
laparoscopy, initial   40–1, 80, 84
laparotomy set   115
laser light
    delivery   33
    properties   29
laser resonator   29, 30

lasers
  Argon 31
  carbon dioxide (CO_2) 31
  characteristics 31–3
  contact 33–4
  continuous-wave mode 30
  dangers associated 31
  energy production 29–30
  interaction with tissues 30–1
  KTP 32
  Neodymium YAG 32
  position 76
  pulsed mode 30
  safety precautions 31
  techniques 45–6
  theoretical background 28–9
lasing media 29, 31–3
laxatives, pre-operative 58
Ligaclip 24
light cable 8, 79
  damage to 109
light source 8
  position 76
linea alba, closing 97–8
lithotripsy 128
  laparoscopic 107
lithotripter forceps 128
lithotripters, ultrasonic/electrostatic
  128
liver, percussion, during initial
    insufflation 39
liver function tests 57–8
Lloyd Davies position, modified 75
lungs, maximal postoperative
    inflation 65

magnetic resonance imaging,
    interference by metal clips 25
mesentery 68
metoclopramide 65
microscissors 16, 17
minimal access surgery xiii
mobility, postoperative 132
monitors 9–10
  positioning 74, 75
muscle relaxation
  intra-operative 63
  loss of 112

nausea, postoperative 66–7
Nd–YAG lasers 32–3
needle holders 20–1

needles
  loss of in peritoneal cavity 124–5
  ski 24
  Verres 1, 2, 37–8, 40
    surgical trauma with 121–2
    testing 80
Nehzat probe 23
neostigmine 63
neodymium–yttrium aluminium garnet
    lasers 32–3
neuromuscular blockade,
    monitoring 63
nitrous oxide, in insufflation 10
non-steroidal anti-inflammatory drugs
  postoperative 66
  pre-operative 61
Novacol 116
NSAIDs
  postoperative 66
  pre-operative 61

obesity, problems associated 61, 81,
    110–11
omentum, pushing/pulling
    downwards 42
open cholecystectomy 100–1
  conversion to 60
operating techniques 80–99
  summary with normal anatomy 69
operating theatre
  layout 74–6
  setting up 76–8
operative difficulties 108–29
opiates 131
optical fibres, broken 8
oral cholecystography, pre-operative
    57
oral feeding, postoperative 132
oral fluids, postoperative intake 131
oro-gastric intubation 65, 131
overblankets 62
oxygen, in insufflation 10

pain
  persistent 130–1
  postoperative 66, 130–1
  shoulder 66, 130
  wound 66, 130
pancreatitis 56, 100
paracetamol 130, 131
past burning 31
patients
  collapse 129

information 60, 100, 134–5
informed consent 60
intra-operative positioning 65,
    74–5
preparation 58–9
safety 65
perforation of gallbladder 123
perforation of bowel (freeing
        adhesions) 121–2
peritoneal toilet 95
peritoneum
    adhesions 116–19
    dividing 42–3, 87
peritonitis 56
Petelin forceps 21–2, 46
Petelin technique
        (cholangiography) 88–90
Petelin's method (choledoscopy)
        106–7
pethidine, postoperative 66
photons, emission 28–9
plain scissors 16, 17
pheumoperitoneum
    dangers associated 40
    loss of 112
    producing 1, 37–8
        problems in obesity 110–11
    safety tests 38–9
polyglactin, as suture material 24
population inversion 29
porta hepatis, access obscured by
        adhesions 118
portal vein, haemorrhage from
        114–15
ports
    exit
        choice of 95
        enlarging 97, 98
    haemorrhage from 112–13
    insertion 80
        first/umbilical 80–1, 84
        second/subcostal 81–2, 84
        third/lateral 82, 83, 84
        fourth/epigastric 82–4
    insertion of extra 42
    positioning 35, 37
positive pressure ventilation 62
postoperative care 130–2
    after bile duct injury 122–3
postoperative sepsis, previous, as
        contraindication 56
potassium titanyl phosphate lasers 32

premedication 59, 61–2, 131
pre-operative management 56–60
    anaesthetic 61–2
printer 10
pyramidal trocar point 3–4

recovery 60
Reddick–Olsen cholangiography
        clamp 26, 90
reducing sleeves/diaphragms 2
retraction
    abdominal wall 41
    falciform ligament 41–2
    gallbladder 41
retractors, fixed 79
retroperitoneal haematoma 40,
        113–14
right hepatic duct, mistaken for cystic
        duct 70, 71
Roeder knot 49–50
    pretied 50–1

safety tests, pneumoperitoneum 38–9
saline, as irrigating fluid 23
saline bag, use as irrigation
        device 22, 23
scissors 16–17
    insulated, blunting 17
    technique 44–5
scrub nurse 76
self-holding devices 17–18
setting up 74–80
severity of disease, assessment 56
shaving, pre-operative 58, 78
shivering, postoperative 67
shoulder pain 66, 130
single jaw mechanism, forceps 20
ski needle 24
skin
    closure 98–9
    preparation 58, 78
smoke
    extraction 11, 12–13, 63, 109
    and loss of vision 109
sphincter of Oddi, dilatation 102–3
sphincterotomy
    endoscopic precholecystectomy 100
    indicators for 56
    pre-operative 58
spinal kyphosis 57
spot size 33
spring-loaded valves, cannulae 1, 3

stereoscopic vision, lack of   35, 37
sterile connections   77, 78–9
sterile towels, application   78
sterilization, camera   9, 79
stone extracting forceps   20, 124
stones
   large   128
   loss of in peritoneum   123–4
subcutaneous cannulation   81
subhepatic biliary collection   131
subhepatic haematoma   131
sucker
   in retrieval of lost stones   124
   in smoke extraction   109
suction
   dangers   47
   technique   47
suction devices   22–3
   connections   78–9
   position   76
superior epigastric artery,
     puncture   84
supra-umbilical incision   38
surgeon, position   74–5
surgical emphysema   40
surgical trauma   121–5
Surgicel   116
suture materials, catgut as   50
sutures   24
   linea alba   97–8
   skin   98–9
suturing
   dangers   53
   technique   52–3
symptoms, atypical, persistence   56
syringe test   38–9

telescopic-grasping mechanism   19
telescopic springs, forceps   18
temazepam   61
temperature monitoring, intra-operative
   62
testing routines   79–80
thread first technique   24
tissues, interaction with lasers   30–1
tracheal intubation   62

trocars   1, 3–4
   shielded   4
   surgical trauma with   121–2
trolleys, arrangements   76
trumpet valve, cannulae   1, 3

ultrasound
   lithotripters   128
   pre-operative   57
Urograffin   90

vacuum test   38
vascular instruments   115
vecuronium   63
vena cava
   penetration   40
   repair   114
venous access, intra-operative   64
venting circuit   11, 63
   checking   12, 109
   input/output line connection   11
   sterile connections   78
Venturi effect   11–12
Verres needle   1, 2, 37–8, 40
   surgical trauma with   121–2
   testing   80
Vicryl   24
video monitors   9–10
   positioning   74, 75
video printer   10
video recorder   10
video system   8–10
video tapes   60
vision, loss of   108–9
Voltarol   59, 61, 130, 131

Wallace piggy back central venous
     catheter   26
warming blankets   62
water blankets   62
white balancing, camera   9
work, return to   132
wound dehiscence, history of   57
wound pain   66, 130

xenon light source   8